# quick
# & easy
# chicken

*Diabetes-Friendly Recipes Everyone Will Love*

LINDA GASSENHEIMER

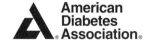
American Diabetes Association®

Director, Book Publishing, Abe Ogden; Managing Editor, Greg Guthrie; Acquisitions Editor, Victor Van Beuren; Project Manager, Boldface LLC; Production Manager, Melissa Sprott; Composition, ADA; Cover Design, Jody Billert; Printer, United Graphics, LLC.

Printed in the United States of America
1 3 5 7 9 10 8 6 4 2

The suggestions and information contained in this publication are generally consistent with the Clinical Practice Recommendations and other policies of the American Diabetes Association, but they do not represent the policy or position of the Association or any of its boards or committees. Reasonable steps have been taken to ensure the accuracy of the information presented. However, the American Diabetes Association cannot ensure the safety or efficacy of any product or service described in this publication. Individuals are advised to consult a physician or other appropriate health care professional before undertaking any diet or exercise program or taking any medication referred to in this publication. Professionals must use and apply their own professional judgment, experience, and training and should not rely solely on the information contained in this publication before prescribing any diet, exercise, or medication. The American Diabetes Association— its officers, directors, employees, volunteers, and members—assumes no responsibility or liability for personal or other injury, loss, or damage that may result from the suggestions or information in this publication.

⊚ The paper in this publication meets the requirements of the ANSI Standard Z39.48-1992 (permanence of paper).

ADA titles may be purchased for business or promotional use or for special sales. To purchase more than 50 copies of this book at a discount, or for custom editions of this book with your logo, contact the American Diabetes Association at the address below, at booksales@diabetes.org, or by calling 703-299-2046.

American Diabetes Association
1701 North Beauregard Street
Alexandria, Virginia 22311

DOI: 10.2337/9781580405638

**Library of Congress Cataloging-in-Publication Data**
Gassenheimer, Linda.
  Quick & easy chicken : diabetes-friendly recipes everyone will love / Linda Gassenheimer.
    pages cm
  title: Quick and easy chicken
  Includes bibliographical references and index.
  ISBN 978-1-58040-563-8 (alk. paper)
  1. Diabetes--Diet therapy--Recipes. 2. Cooking (Chicken) 3. Quick and easy cooking. 4. International cooking. I. Title. II. Title: Quick and easy chicken.
  RC662.G39 2015
  641.5'6314--dc23

                    2014025361

To my husband, Harold,
for his love,
constant enthusiasm for my work,
and support.

# Contents

# Acknowledgments

One of the best parts of writing a book is working with so many talented and friendly people. I'd like to thank them all for their enthusiastic support.

My biggest thank-you goes to my husband, Harold, who supported me, helped me test every recipe, and spent hours helping me edit every word. His constant encouragement of all of my work has made this book a partnership.

Thank you to Abe Ogden, director of book publishing at the American Diabetes Association, for his guidance and support. He worked closely with me to bring this book to life.

Thank you to Joseph Cooper and Bonnie Berman, hosts of *Topical Currents*, and to the staff at WLRN National Public Radio for their help and enthusiasm for my weekly "Food News and Views" segment.

I'd also like to thank my family, who have supported my projects and encouraged me every step of the way: my son James, his wife, Patty, and their children, Zachary, Jacob, and Haley; my son John, his wife, Jill, and their children, Jeffrey and Joanna; my son Charles, his wife, Lori, and their sons, Daniel and Matthew; and my sister, Roberta, and her husband, Robert.

And, finally, thank you to all of my readers and listeners who have written and called over the years. You have helped to shape my ideas and have made the solitary task of writing a two-way street.

# Introduction

Throughout history, chicken dishes have been a symbol of comfort and well-being. Henry IV, the king of France, wanted no peasant to be without a chicken in his pot every Sunday. Franklin Roosevelt's 1932 party slogan was "two chickens in every pot." Today, as then, chicken is a staple of hearty, healthy meals.

Grilled, sautéed, roasted, or poached—chicken is a great palette to paint a meal on. From All-American to Asian, African, Latin American, or Mediterranean dishes, chicken is the perfect meat to carry these flavors. You'll find a wide range of dishes to fit your every mood in this book. The recipes are quick, easy, and family-friendly.

Feeling like American comfort food? Try the Sangria-Braised Pulled Chicken Sliders or the Pecan-Crusted, Honey-Glazed Chicken. Enjoy a hint of India with Curry-Kissed Chicken or a Chinese dinner with Kung Pao Chicken. Or savor the flavors of North Africa with Moroccan Spiced Chicken. Looking for a soup supper? The Garlic-Chicken Soup with Sesame-Parmesan Crostini might fit the bill. And for those times when you want a quick sandwich meal, make the Barbecued-Chicken Roll or Sloppy Joes.

All of the recipes are complete meals based on ingredients you can easily find in your local supermarket. Look at the Shop Smart section of this book (page xi) for help choosing the right ingredients.

For ease and speed, all of these recipes use chicken parts rather than whole chickens.

## Helpful Hints and Countdown

Each recipe contains tips on shopping and cooking and a game plan (countdown), so you can get the whole meal on the table at the same time.

## Shopping

Many staple ingredients are used throughout this book. If you keep these staple items on hand, you'll only need to pick up the fresh ingredients to make delicious meals in minutes.

- Oils: olive oil, olive oil cooking spray, vegetable oil cooking spray, canola oil
- Frozen ingredients: frozen diced onion, frozen diced green bell pepper, frozen corn kernels
- Condiments: reduced-fat oil and vinegar dressing, reduced-fat mayonnaise, balsamic vinegar
- Sauces: low-sodium tomato sauce, low-sodium pasta sauce, hot pepper sauce
- Fat-free, low-sodium chicken stock
- Vegetables: minced garlic, whole garlic, carrots, onion
- Spices and herbs (less than 6 months old): ground cumin, dried oregano, dried thyme
- Grains: microwave brown, white, and long-grain white rice

## Chicken Cooking and Storing Tips

### Cooking Temperatures

- Boneless white meat should reach 165°F.
- Boneless dark meat should reach 170°F.
- Juices should be clear, not pink, when pierced by a fork.
- Chicken should never be served medium or rare.

### Storing Chicken

Refrigerate raw chicken immediately. It should not be stored at room temperature.

Freeze uncooked chicken if it is not used within 2 days.

### Thawing Frozen Chicken

Always thaw chicken in the refrigerator. Cut-up parts will take about 3–9 hours to thaw.

For quick thawing, place the chicken (wrapped well) in cold water and change the water often.

### Safety

Wash hands, countertops, cutting boards, knives, and other utensils used in preparing raw chicken with soapy hot water.

# Shop Smart

To help make these dinners in minutes, I have used ingredients you can find in your local supermarket. This guide isn't a specific recommendation of any particular brand. You can choose from the many options available. The key is to shop smart by looking at the nutrition information provided in this section. I have listed the items for which I have found a range of products with variations in calorie, fat, carbohydrate, or sodium content to guide you toward healthy options. You may not find the exact values. Use this information as a guideline for what you choose. Once you find ingredients you like, keep them on hand so that you only have to shop for a few fresh ingredients.

Look for the following:

- Fat-free, low-sodium chicken stock or broth with 20 calories per cup and about 150 mg sodium per cup.

- Low-sodium pasta sauce with 130 calories, less than 4.0 g fat, and 80 mg sodium per cup.

- Low-sodium tomato sauce with 70 calories, 0.5 g fat, and 27 mg sodium per cup.

- Low-sodium, no-sugar-added, diced tomatoes with 41 calories, 0.3 g fat, 0.04 g saturated fat, and 24 mg sodium per cup.

- Light coconut milk with 150 calories, 12.0 g fat, and 45 mg sodium per cup.

- Light tortillas, 8–9 inches in diameter, weighing 39 g (or 1 1/2 ounces), with 80 calories, 2.0 g fat, and 250 mg sodium per tortilla.

- Corn tortillas, 6 inches in diameter, weighing 26 g (a little under 1 ounce), with 58 calories, 7.0 g fat, and 3 mg sodium per tortilla.

- Whole-wheat tortillas, 8 inches in diameter, weighing 48 g (a little under 2 ounces), with 130 calories, 2 g fat, and 330 mg sodium per tortilla.

- Whole-wheat pita breads, about 6 inches in diameter, weighing 64 g (a little over 2 ounces), with 170 calories, 1.7 g fat, and 284 mg sodium each.

- Canned fat-free refried beans with 182 calories, 1.0 g fat, and 1012 mg sodium per cup.

- Chimichurri sauce with 90 calories, 9.5 g fat, and 33 mg sodium per tablespoon (Example: Badia Chimichurri Steak Sauce).

- Ground chicken made from chicken breast meat only. If the label just says "ground chicken," then skin, fat, and dark meat may have been added.

- Low-sodium ketchup with 16 calories and 3 mg sodium per tablespoon.

# All-American

# Almond-Maple Chicken with Hot Pepper Succotash

*A maple syrup glaze and sliced almonds give extra flavor and crunch to chicken breasts. Hot pepper jelly adds zing to sautéed corn and lima beans. The Hot Pepper Succotash can be made in minutes in the microwave.*

## Countdown:

- Place succotash in microwave.
- While succotash cooks, make chicken dish.

## Almond-Maple Chicken

Serves: 2 / Serving Size: 5 ounces chicken, 1 tablespoon sauce

> 3/4 pound boneless, skinless chicken breasts
> 2 tablespoons maple syrup
> 1 tablespoon canola oil
> Olive oil cooking spray
> Salt and freshly ground black pepper, to taste
> 2 tablespoons sliced almonds

1. Remove all visible fat from chicken.

2. Mix maple syrup and canola oil together. Set aside.

3. Heat a nonstick skillet, just big enough to hold chicken in one layer, over medium-high heat. Spray skillet with olive oil cooking spray, add chicken, and cover with a lid. Sauté 5 minutes. Turn and sauté, covered, 3 more minutes. A meat thermometer inserted into chicken should read 165°F.

4. Remove skillet from heat and pour maple syrup mixture over chicken. Turn chicken over in the sauce and divide chicken between 2 dinner plates.

5. Pour remaining sauce over chicken. Add salt and pepper to taste. Sprinkle almonds on top.

*Exchanges/Food Choices: 1 other carbohydrate, 6 lean protein, 3 fat*
*Per serving: Calories 470, Calories from Fat 230, Total Fat 25 g, Saturated Fat 2.5 g, Monounsaturated Fat 14 g, Cholesterol 125 mg, Sodium 85 mg, Potassium 780 mg, Total Carbohydrate 19 g, Dietary Fiber 3 g, Sugars 15 g, Protein 43 g, Phosphorus 470 mg*

## Hot Pepper Succotash

Serves: 2 / Serving Size: 3/4 cup

**2 tablespoons hot pepper jelly**
**3/4 cup frozen corn kernels**
**3/4 cup frozen lima beans**

1. Place all ingredients in a microwave-safe bowl. Cover with a plate or plastic wrap.

2. Microwave on high 2 minutes.

3. Toss well and serve.

**Stove-top Method:** Place hot pepper jelly, corn, and lima beans in a skillet over medium-high heat. Sauté 3 minutes. The vegetables only need to be warmed through.

*Exchanges/Food Choices: 2 starch, 1/2 other carbohydrate*
*Per serving: Calories 180, Calories from Fat 5, Total Fat 0.5 g, Saturated Fat 0 g,*
*Monounsaturated Fat 0 g, Cholesterol 0 mg, Sodium 40 mg, Potassium 400 mg,*
*Total Carbohydrate 41 g, Dietary Fiber 5 g, Sugars 13 g, Protein 6 g, Phosphorus 100 mg*

## Shopping List:

3/4 pound boneless, skinless chicken breasts
1 bottle maple syrup
1 small package sliced almonds
1 jar hot pepper jelly
1 package frozen corn kernels
1 package frozen lima beans

## Staples:

Canola oil
Olive oil cooking spray
Salt and black peppercorns

## Helpful Hints:

- Walnuts, pistachios, or pecans can be substituted for sliced almonds.
- Any type of hot pepper jelly can be used.

# Cajun Chicken with Caramelized Onion Rice

*Cajun cooking is considered the country cousin to Creole cuisine.
Cajun is often referred to as country food. It's hot and spicy. If you like
your food really hot, serve hot pepper sauce on the side.*

## Countdown:

- Marinate chicken.
- Start cooking onions and red bell pepper.
- Remove to a bowl and use same skillet for chicken.
- Make chicken.
- Finish rice.

## Cajun Chicken

Serves: 2 / Serving Size: 5 ounces chicken

> 3/4 pound boneless, skinless chicken breasts
> 1/2 teaspoon paprika
> 1/2 teaspoon black pepper
> 1/4 teaspoon cayenne pepper
> 1/2 teaspoon dried thyme
> 1/8 teaspoon salt
> 1/2 teaspoon garlic powder
> 2 teaspoons canola oil

1. Place chicken between 2 pieces of plastic wrap and pound it to an even thickness of about 1/2 inch.

2. Mix paprika, black pepper, cayenne pepper, dried thyme, salt, and garlic powder together in a bowl. Add chicken to the seasoning mix and roll, being sure to coat both sides. Set aside while preparing remaining ingredients for the meal.

3. Heat oil over medium heat in the nonstick skillet used to cook the onions. Add chicken to skillet and sauté 2 minutes. Turn and sauté 2 minutes. Remove from heat, cover with a lid, and let sit 10 minutes. (Cook 3 minutes per side for 1-inch-thick pieces of chicken.) A meat thermometer inserted into cooked chicken should read 165°F.

*Exchanges/Food Choices: 5 lean protein, 1/2 fat*
*Per serving: Calories 250, Calories from Fat 80, Total Fat 9 g, Saturated Fat 1.5 g,*
*Monounsaturated Fat 4 g, Cholesterol 125 mg, Sodium 220 mg, Potassium 600 mg,*
*Total Carbohydrate 2 g, Dietary Fiber <1 g, Sugars 0 g, Protein 39 g, Phosphorus 365 mg*

# Caramelized Onion Rice

Serves: 2 / Serving Size: 1 3/4 cups rice/vegetable mixture

> 2 cups sliced onion
> 2 teaspoons canola oil
> 1 cup sliced red bell pepper
> Salt and freshly ground black pepper, to taste
> 1 package microwave brown rice (to yield at least 1 1/2 cups cooked rice)

1. Place onion in a microwave-safe bowl and microwave on high 5 minutes.

2. Heat oil in a nonstick skillet over medium-high heat. Add the onions and red bell pepper. Sauté 5 minutes, stirring during that time. Add salt and pepper to taste. Remove to a bowl.

3. Cook rice according to package instructions. Measure out 1 1/2 cups rice and set aside any remaining rice for another meal.

4. Add rice to the bowl with the onions and red bell pepper. Toss well.

*Exchanges/Food Choices: 2 1/2 starch, 1 vegetable, 1 fat*
*Per serving: Calories 270, Calories from Fat 45, Total Fat 5 g, Saturated Fat 0.5 g,*
*Monounsaturated Fat 3 g, Cholesterol 0 mg, Sodium 10 mg, Potassium 320 mg,*
*Total Carbohydrate 51 g, Dietary Fiber 4 g, Sugars 7 g, Protein 5 g, Phosphorus 100 mg*

## Shopping List:

3/4 pound boneless, skinless chicken breasts
1 bottle paprika
1 bottle cayenne pepper
1 bottle dried thyme
1 bottle garlic powder
1 red bell pepper
1 package microwave brown rice

## Staples:

Salt and black peppercorns
Canola oil
Onion

## Helpful Hints:

- Any type of onion can be used.
- Spread seasonings over chicken and let stand while preparing the remaining ingredients and rice.
- Sauté chicken on a low flame to keep the spices from burning.
- Make sure your bottles of dried herbs and spices are less than 6 months old.

# Chicken in Sherry-Mushroom Sauce with Herbed Quinoa

*Slow cooking in sherry produces a moist, tender, and flavorful chicken dinner. Mushrooms add an earthiness to this dish. It can be made ahead of time and rewarmed.*

## Countdown:

- Start cooking chicken.
- While chicken cooks, make quinoa.
- Complete chicken dish.

### Chicken in Sherry-Mushroom Sauce

Serves: 2 / Serving Size: 5 ounces chicken, 1 cup vegetables, 2 tablespoons sauce

> 1 1/2 pounds skinless chicken legs with bone
> 1/2 lemon
> 2 teaspoons olive oil
> 2 teaspoons minced garlic
> 1 cup dry sherry
> 1/2 pound sliced Portobello mushrooms
> Salt and freshly ground black pepper, to taste

1. Rub the chicken with the half lemon.

2. In a nonstick skillet just large enough to hold the legs in one layer, heat oil over medium-high heat.

3. Add the chicken legs and brown 2 minutes. Turn and brown 2 more minutes.

4. Reduce the heat to low, and add the garlic and sherry. Cover tightly and cook 10 minutes, turning from time to time.

5. Add the mushrooms to the chicken and cook, uncovered, 5 minutes. A meat thermometer inserted into chicken should read 170°F. Add salt and pepper to taste.

*Exchanges/Food Choices: 1 other carbohydrate, 1 vegetable, 5 1/2 lean protein, 2 fat*
*Per serving: Calories 460, Calories from Fat 110, Total Fat 12 g, Saturated Fat 2.5 g,*
*Monounsaturated Fat 6 g, Cholesterol 160 mg, Sodium 180 mg, Potassium 930 mg,*
*Total Carbohydrate 20 g, Dietary Fiber 1 g, Sugars 4 g, Protein 38 g, Phosphorus 435 mg*

## Herbed Quinoa

Serves: 2 / Serving Size: 3/4 cup

> 1/2 cup quinoa
> 2 cups water
> 1/4 cup chopped parsley
> 1/4 cup sliced chives
> 1 teaspoon olive oil
> Salt and freshly ground black pepper, to taste

1. Place quinoa in a colander or sieve with small openings and run cold water over the grains. Let drain.

2. Place the quinoa and water in a saucepan. Bring to a boil over high heat.

3. Reduce heat to medium, cover with a lid, and cook 10 minutes. All of the water should be absorbed. If the pan runs dry before the quinoa is cooked, add more water.

4. Add the parsley, chives, olive oil, and salt and pepper. Place quinoa on a plate, and serve chicken and sauce on top.

*Exchanges/Food Choices: 2 starch, 1/2 fat*
*Per serving: Calories 180, Calories from Fat 45, Total Fat 5 g, Saturated Fat 0.5 g,*
*Monounsaturated Fat 2.5 g, Cholesterol 0 mg, Sodium 5 mg, Potassium 300 mg,*
*Total Carbohydrate 28 g, Dietary Fiber 3 g, Sugars 0 g, Protein 6 g, Phosphorus 205 mg*

## Shopping List:

1 1/2 pounds skinless chicken legs with bone
1 lemon
1 bottle dry sherry
1 package sliced Portobello mushrooms (1/2 pound needed)
1 package quinoa
1 bunch parsley
1 bunch chives

## Staples:

Olive oil
Minced garlic
Salt and black peppercorns

## Helpful Hints:

- Any type of mushroom can be used.
- Sherry should be cooked over a low heat. It burns easily.
- The skillet should be just large enough to hold the chicken legs in one layer. If it is too big, the juices will run along the bottom and evaporate.
- A quick way to chop parsley and chives is to snip them with a scissors.

# Chicken in Red Wine with Parsley Noodles

*Chicken cooked in a rich red wine sauce is a French classic. This quick
version captures the French flavors without all the fuss.*

## Countdown:

- Place water for noodles on to boil.
- Start chicken.
- Make noodles.
- Complete chicken dish.

### Chicken in Red Wine

Serves: 2 / Serving Size: 5 ounces chicken, 2 cups vegetables, 1/4 cup sauce

2 teaspoons canola oil
1 1/2 pounds skinless chicken legs
  with bone
1 cup sliced onion
1 cup sliced carrots
1 teaspoon minced garlic
2 tablespoons water

1/2 cup red wine
1/2 cup fat-free, low-sodium
  chicken stock
1/2 pound button mushrooms, cut
  into quarters
Salt and freshly ground black
  pepper, to taste

1. In a nonstick skillet just large enough to hold the chicken legs in one layer, heat oil over medium-high heat.

2. Add the chicken, onion, carrots, and minced garlic. Brown the chicken on all sides, and stir vegetables for about 5 minutes.

3. Add water, reduce heat to medium, and cover with a lid. Cook 10 minutes. A meat thermometer inserted into chicken should read 170°F. Remove chicken and vegetables to a plate.

4. Raise the heat to high and add the wine to the skillet, scraping up the brown bits on the bottom of the skillet. Reduce the wine by half (about 4–5 minutes), and add the chicken stock and mushrooms. Simmer 3–4 minutes. Return the chicken and vegetables to the skillet to warm through.

5. Sprinkle with salt and pepper to taste. Serve over the noodles.

*Exchanges/Food Choices: 3 vegetable, 5 1/2 lean protein, 1 fat
Per serving: Calories 370, Calories from Fat 110, Total Fat 12 g, Saturated Fat 2.5 g,
Monounsaturated Fat 5 g, Cholesterol 160 mg, Sodium 250 mg, Potassium 1210 mg,
Total Carbohydrate 17 g, Dietary Fiber 4 g, Sugars 8 g, Protein 40 g, Phosphorus 500 mg*

## Parsley Noodles

Serves: 2 / Serving Size: 3/4 cup

> 1/4 pound fresh whole-wheat linguine
> 1/4 cup chopped parsley
> 2 teaspoons canola oil
> Salt and freshly ground black pepper, to taste

1. Bring a large pot with 3–4 quarts water to a boil.

2. Add the linguine. Boil 2–3 minutes or until tender but firm.

3. Place parsley in a mixing bowl and add the oil and 1 tablespoon pasta cooking water. Drain the pasta and add to the bowl.

4. Toss until pasta is coated with the parsley. Add salt and pepper to taste.

*Exchanges/Food Choices: 3 starch, 1 fat*
*Per serving: Calories 250, Calories from Fat 45, Total Fat 5 g, Saturated Fat 0.5 g,*
*Monounsaturated Fat 3 g, Cholesterol 0 mg, Sodium 5 mg, Potassium 170 mg,*
*Total Carbohydrate 43 g, Dietary Fiber 2 g, Sugars 2 g, Protein 8 g, Phosphorus 110 mg*

## Shopping List:

1 1/2 pounds skinless chicken legs with bone
1 bottle red wine
1 package button mushrooms (1/2 pound needed)
1 package fresh whole-wheat linguine
1 bunch parsley

## Staples:

Canola oil
Onion
Carrots
Minced garlic
Fat-free, low-sodium chicken stock
Salt and black peppercorns

## Helpful Hints:

- Look for skinless chicken legs with the bone, or remove the skin before cooking.
- Dried linguine can be used instead of fresh. Boil dried linguine for 10 minutes.
- A quick way to chop parsley is to snip the leaves from the stems with a scissors.
- Any type of onion can be used.

## Shop Smart:

- Look for fat-free, low-sodium chicken stock or broth with 20 calories per cup and about 150 mg sodium per cup.

# Creole Chicken with Brown Rice

*Green pepper, celery, and onions are essential ingredients in Creole and Cajun cooking. Add pasta sauce, hot peppers, and chicken, and you've got a quick and easy Chicken Creole.*

## Countdown:

- Make rice and set aside.
- Make chicken.

## Creole Chicken

Serves: 2 / Serving Size: 5 ounces chicken, 2 cups vegetables, 1/2 cup sauce

> 2 teaspoons olive oil
> 3/4 pound boneless, skinless chicken breasts, cut into 1-inch cubes
> 1 cup sliced onion
> 1 cup sliced green bell pepper
> 1 cup sliced celery
> 2 teaspoons minced garlic
> 1 1/4 cups low-sodium pasta sauce
> 1 tablespoon Worcestershire sauce
> 1/8 teaspoon cayenne pepper
> Salt and freshly ground black pepper, to taste
> Hot pepper sauce, to taste

1. Heat olive oil in a medium-size nonstick skillet over high heat. Add chicken cubes and brown on all sides for 3 minutes.

2. Remove chicken to a plate and reduce heat under skillet to medium high. Add onion, green pepper, celery, and garlic to skillet, and sauté 3 minutes.

3. Add pasta sauce, Worcestershire sauce, and cayenne pepper, and return chicken to skillet. Stir to combine ingredients. Simmer 3 minutes. A meat thermometer inserted into chicken should read 165°F.

4. Add salt and pepper to taste. Spoon chicken and sauce over rice, and add hot pepper sauce to taste.

*Exchanges/Food Choices: 4 vegetable, 6 lean protein*
*Per serving: Calories 380, Calories from Fat 110, Total Fat 12 g, Saturated Fat 2 g,*
*Monounsaturated Fat 5 g, Cholesterol 130 mg, Sodium 260 mg, Potassium 1470 mg,*
*Total Carbohydrate 26 g, Dietary Fiber 6 g, Sugars 14 g, Protein 42 g, Phosphorus 465 mg*

## Brown Rice

Serves: 2 / Serving Size: 3/4 cup

> 1 package microwave brown rice
>   (to yield at least 1 1/2 cups cooked rice)
> 2 teaspoons olive oil
> Salt and freshly ground black pepper, to taste

1. Cook rice according to package instructions. Measure out 1 1/2 cups rice and set aside any remaining rice for another meal.

2. Add the olive oil and salt and pepper to taste. Serve with the chicken.

*Exchanges/Food Choices: 2 starch, 1 fat*
*Per serving: Calories 200, Calories from Fat 50, Total Fat 6 g, Saturated Fat 1 g,*
*Monounsaturated Fat 4 g, Cholesterol 0 mg, Sodium 10 mg, Potassium 65 mg,*
*Total Carbohydrate 34 g, Dietary Fiber 3 g, Sugars <1 g, Protein 4 g, Phosphorus 120 mg*

## Shopping List:

3/4 pound boneless, skinless chicken
    breasts
1 green bell pepper
1 bunch celery
1 can low-sodium pasta sauce
1 bottle Worcestershire sauce
1 bottle cayenne pepper
1 bottle hot pepper sauce
1 package microwave brown rice

## Staples:

Olive oil
Onion
Minced garlic
Salt and black peppercorns

## Helpful Hints:

■ Minced garlic can be found in the produce section of the market.
■ Any type of onion can be used.

## Shop Smart:

■ Look for low-sodium pasta sauce with 130 calories, less than 4 g fat, and 80 mg sodium per cup.

# Devil's Chicken with Sautéed Garlic Potatoes

*Two types of strong, flavorful mustards give the sauce for this sautéed chicken its character. It's a version of a typical French bistro dish. Potatoes cooked with garlic add another French-inspired touch.*

## Countdown:

- Microwave potatoes and set aside.
- Make chicken.
- Remove chicken from skillet and add potatoes.

### Devil's Chicken

Serves: 2 / Serving Size: 5 ounces chicken, 1 cup vegetables, 2 tablespoons sauce

> 2 tablespoons flour
> Salt and freshly ground black pepper, to taste
> 3/4 pound boneless, skinless chicken breasts
> 2 teaspoons canola oil
> 1/4 cup dry vermouth
> 1 tablespoon Dijon mustard
> 1 tablespoon coarse-grain mustard
> 1/4 cup water
> 1/2 pound green beans, cut into 2-inch pieces
> 1 tablespoon light cream

1. Place flour on a plate and sprinkle with salt and pepper to taste. Add chicken and roll in the flour, making sure both sides of each breast are covered. Shake off the excess.

2. Heat oil in a nonstick skillet over medium-high heat. Add chicken and brown for 3 minutes. Turn and brown second side for 3 minutes. Add vermouth and cook 1 minute.

3. In a small bowl, blend mustards with water and add to skillet. Bring liquid to a simmer, scraping up browned bits in the pan.

4. Reduce heat to medium, add green beans, cover, and gently simmer 5 minutes. A meat thermometer inserted into chicken should read 165°F.

5. Remove chicken to 2 dinner plates.

6. Add cream to the skillet and stir to mix well. Spoon sauce over chicken. Reserve skillet for potatoes.

*Exchanges/Food Choices: 2 vegetable, 6 lean protein, 1/2 fat*
*Per serving: Calories 340, Calories from Fat 100, Total Fat 11 g, Saturated Fat 2.5 g,*
*Monounsaturated Fat 5 g, Cholesterol 130 mg, Sodium 460 mg, Potassium 850 mg,*
*Total Carbohydrate 12 g, Dietary Fiber 4 g, Sugars 4 g, Protein 42 g, Phosphorus 430 mg*

## Sautéed Garlic Potatoes

Serves: 2 / Serving Size: 1 cup

> 1 pound red potatoes, unpeeled, washed, and cut into 1-inch pieces
> 3 large garlic cloves, unpeeled
> 2 teaspoons canola oil
> Salt and freshly ground black pepper, to taste

1. Place potatoes in a microwave-safe bowl and microwave on high 5 minutes.
2. Remove from microwave and add garlic cloves. Set aside.
3. After chicken is removed from the skillet, add canola oil and turn heat to high.
4. Add the potatoes and garlic to skillet. Sauté the potatoes for about 5 minutes to brown on all sides. Remove garlic and serve potatoes with the chicken.

*Exchanges/Food Choices: 2 starch, 1 fat*
*Per serving: Calories 200, Calories from Fat 45, Total Fat 5 g, Saturated Fat 0 g,*
*Monounsaturated Fat 3 g, Cholesterol 0 mg, Sodium 40 mg, Potassium 1030 mg,*
*Total Carbohydrate 36 g, Dietary Fiber 4 g, Sugars 3 g, Protein 4 g, Phosphorus 140 mg*

## Shopping List:

- 3/4 pound boneless, skinless chicken breasts
- 1 small bottle dry vermouth
- 1 jar Dijon mustard
- 1 jar coarse-grain mustard
- 1 package green beans (1/2 pound needed)
- 1 small carton light cream
- 1 pound red potatoes

## Staples:

Flour
Salt and black peppercorns
Canola oil
Garlic

## Helpful Hints:

■ Trimmed green beans can be found in the produce section of the market.
■ Use a skillet just large enough to hold the chicken. If the skillet is too large, the sauce will evaporate.

# Dilled Chicken Parcels with Parsley Rice

*When chicken topped with vegetables and dill is cooked in a parcel, the natural flavor is sealed into the parcel. The chicken is succulent, and the vegetables are cooked just right. The secret is to make sure your oven is at temperature when adding the parcels.*

## Countdown:

- Preheat oven to 450°F.
- Prepare chicken parcels.
- While chicken cooks, make rice dish.

### Dilled Chicken Parcels

Serves: 2 / Serving Size: 5 ounces chicken, 1 cup vegetables, 2 tablespoons sauce

> 2 circles of aluminum foil or parchment paper (about 12 inches in diameter)
> 2 teaspoons olive oil
> 3/4 pound boneless, skinless chicken breast cutlets,
>     thinly sliced into 1/4-inch-thick slices
> 2 tablespoons chopped fresh dill OR 2 teaspoons dried dill
> Salt and freshly ground black pepper, to taste
> 1 cup frozen diced onion, defrosted
> 1 cup frozen diced green peppers, defrosted
> 1 1/4 cups thinly sliced Portobello mushrooms
> 1/4 cup dry white wine

1. Preheat oven to 450°F.

2. Coat one half of each paper or foil circle with olive oil. Divide the chicken in half and place half on the oiled part of each circle.

3. Sprinkle half the dill over chicken in each parcel along with salt and pepper to taste. Spoon half of the onion, green pepper, and mushrooms into each parcel. Spoon 2 tablespoons wine into each parcel.

4. Close the parcels by folding the empty half over the half that contains the chicken and sealing the edges. If using foil, bend the edges over and press together. If using parchment paper, fold the edges together and then fold them around the semi-circle, overlapping the previous fold as you go.

5. Place on a baking tray and bake 15 minutes. A meat thermometer inserted into chicken should read 165°F.

6. To serve, place each parcel on an individual plate and open at the table.

Or lift the chicken and vegetables out of the parcels onto each plate and pour the sauce over them.

*Exchanges/Food Choices: 2 vegetable, 5 1/2 lean protein, 1/2 fat*
*Per serving: Calories 310, Calories from Fat 80, Total Fat 9 g, Saturated Fat 1.5 g,*
*Monounsaturated Fat 4.5 g, Cholesterol 125 mg, Sodium 95 mg, Potassium 920 mg,*
*Total Carbohydrate 10 g, Dietary Fiber 3 g, Sugars 5 g, Protein 41 g, Phosphorus 430 mg*

## Parsley Rice

Serves: 2 / Serving Size: 3/4 cup

**1 package microwave brown rice**
   **(to yield at least 1 1/2 cups cooked rice)**
**1/4 cup chopped parsley**
**2 teaspoons olive oil**
**Salt and freshly ground black pepper, to taste**

1. Cook rice according to package instructions. Measure out 1 1/2 cups and set aside any remaining rice for another meal.

2. Add the parsley, olive oil, and salt and pepper to taste.

*Exchanges/Food Choices: 2 starch, 1 fat*
*Per serving: Calories 210, Calories from Fat 50, Total Fat 6 g, Saturated Fat 1 g,*
*Monounsaturated Fat 4 g, Cholesterol 0 mg, Sodium 10 mg, Potassium 105 mg,*
*Total Carbohydrate 34 g, Dietary Fiber 3 g, Sugars <1 g, Protein 4 g, Phosphorus 125 mg*

## Shopping List:

Aluminum foil or parchment paper
3/4 pound boneless, skinless chicken
   breast cutlets
1 bunch fresh or 1 bottle dried dill
1 package frozen diced onion
1 package frozen diced green peppers
1 container sliced Portobello mushrooms
1 bottle dry white wine
1 package microwave brown rice
1 bunch parsley

## Staples:

Olive oil
Salt and black peppercorns

## Helpful Hints:

■ A quick way to chop dill and parsley is to snip the leaves with a scissors.
■ A quick way to defrost the onion and green peppers is to place them in a sieve and run hot tap water over them. Squeeze out extra liquid.

# Fresh Herbed Chicken with Red Potatoes and Green Beans

*Fresh herbs give a fragrant flavor to chicken. With the help of a food processor and microwave oven, this dinner takes only minutes to make. Fresh tarragon has an anise or licorice flavor—if you prefer, use basil, cilantro, or dill instead.*

## Countdown:

- Prepare ingredients.
- Start cooking chicken.
- While chicken cooks, make potatoes and green beans.

### Fresh Herbed Chicken

Serves: 2 / Serving Size: 5 ounces chicken

3 teaspoons olive oil, divided
2 6-ounce boneless, skinless
    chicken breasts
2 tablespoons fresh OR 2
    teaspoons dried tarragon
1/2 cup fresh parsley

3 medium button mushrooms,
    chopped (about 1/2 cup)
1 teaspoon minced garlic
Salt and freshly ground black
    pepper, to taste

1. Heat 1 teaspoon olive oil in a nonstick skillet over medium-high heat.

2. Add the chicken and brown 2 minutes. Turn over and brown 2 more minutes.

3. Reduce heat to medium, cover with a lid, and cook 5 minutes. A meat thermometer inserted into chicken should read 165°F.

4. In a food processor or by hand, coarsely chop the tarragon, parsley, mushrooms, and garlic together.

5. Remove chicken from skillet to 2 dinner plates.

6. Add the remaining 2 teaspoons olive oil to the skillet along with the chopped herbs and garlic. Toss to warm through, about 1 minute. Spoon over the chicken.

*Exchanges/Food Choices: 5 1/2 lean protein, 1 fat*
*Per serving: Calories 280, Calories from Fat 100, Total Fat 11 g, Saturated Fat 2 g,*
*Monounsaturated Fat 6 g, Cholesterol 125 mg, Sodium 90 mg, Potassium 730 mg,*
*Total Carbohydrate 3 g, Dietary Fiber <1 g, Sugars <1 g, Protein 40 g, Phosphorus 390 mg*

## Red Potatoes and Green Beans

Serves: 2 / Serving Size: 1 cup vegetables, 1 cup potatoes

**1 pound red potatoes**
**1/2 pound green beans, trimmed**
**2 teaspoons olive oil**
**Salt and freshly ground black pepper, to taste**

1. Wash but do not peel the potatoes. Thinly slice the potatoes. Cut the slices in half if they are large. Place in a microwave-safe bowl.

2. Cut the green beans in half and add to the bowl. Cover with a plate or plastic wrap and microwave on high 5 minutes.

3. Remove from microwave; test potatoes to see if they are cooked. (Cook for another minute in the microwave if needed.)

4. Place on dinner plates with chicken. Drizzle with olive oil, and add salt and pepper to taste.

*Exchanges/Food Choices: 2 starch, 2 vegetable, 1 fat*
*Per serving: Calories 230, Calories from Fat 45, Total Fat 5 g, Saturated Fat 1 g,*
*Monounsaturated Fat 3.5 g, Cholesterol 0 mg, Sodium 50 mg, Potassium 1270 mg,*
*Total Carbohydrate 44 g, Dietary Fiber 7 g, Sugars 7 g, Protein 6 g, Phosphorus 180 mg*

## Shopping List:

2 6-ounce boneless, skinless chicken breasts
1 bunch fresh tarragon or 1 bottle dried
1 bunch parsley
1 container button mushrooms
1 pound red potatoes
1 1/2-pound package green beans

## Staples:

Olive oil
Minced garlic
Salt and black peppercorns

## Helpful Hints:

■ Any type of waxy potatoes, such as gold or yellow, can be used.
■ Dried tarragon can be used instead of fresh; use 2 teaspoons.
■ Trimmed green beans can be found in the produce section of the market.

# Horseradish-Encrusted Chicken with Garlic Sweet Potatoes and Sugar Snap Peas

*Horseradish mixed with mayonnaise gives a zip to these boneless, skinless chicken thighs, and the panko bread crumbs form a golden crust. Panko bread crumbs are a Japanese variety of bread crumbs that are made from bread that has been baked or toasted, giving them a firm texture.*

## Countdown:

- Prepare ingredients.
- Make chicken.
- While chicken cooks, make potatoes and snap peas.

## Horseradish-Encrusted Chicken

Serves: 2 / Serving Size: 5 ounces chicken

> 3/4 pound boneless, skinless chicken thighs
> 3 tablespoons reduced-fat mayonnaise
> 4 tablespoons prepared horseradish
> 1/4 cup panko bread crumbs
> Olive oil cooking spray
> Salt and freshly ground black pepper, to taste

1. Remove visible fat from the chicken.

2. Mix mayonnaise and horseradish together in a bowl. Place bread crumbs on a plate. Dip chicken into the mayonnaise mixture, making sure all sides are coated. Then dip chicken into bread crumbs, coating all sides. Shake off excess.

3. Heat a large nonstick skillet over medium heat and spray with olive oil cooking spray.

4. Add chicken. Cook 5 minutes, turn, and cook 5 more minutes. A meat thermometer inserted into chicken should read 170°F.

5. Remove to 2 dinner plates and sprinkle with salt and pepper to taste.

*Exchanges/Food Choices: 1/2 starch, 5 lean protein, 1 1/2 fat*
*Per serving: Calories 350, Calories from Fat 150, Total Fat 17 g, Saturated Fat 3 g,*
*Monounsaturated Fat 6 g, Cholesterol 160 mg, Sodium 530 mg, Potassium 520 mg,*
*Total Carbohydrate 13 g, Dietary Fiber 2 g, Sugars 4 g, Protein 35 g, Phosphorus 340 mg*

## Garlic Sweet Potatoes and Sugar Snap Peas

Serves: 2 / Serving Size: 1 cup vegetables

> 1/2 pound sweet potatoes
> 2 cups sugar snap peas (about 6 ounces)
> 1 teaspoon minced garlic
> 1 teaspoon olive oil
> Salt and freshly ground black pepper, to taste

1. Peel potatoes and cut into strips about the same size as the sugar snap peas (about 2 inches x 1/2 inch).

2. Place potatoes, sugar snap peas, and garlic in a microwave-safe bowl. Cover with a plate or plastic wrap. Microwave on high for 3–4 minutes. Potatoes should be cooked through.

3. Add olive oil and salt and pepper. Toss well and serve with chicken.

**Stove-top Method:** Bring a saucepan of water to a boil and add the potatoes. Boil 3 minutes, and add sugar snap peas and garlic. Boil 2 more minutes. Drain. Add olive oil, salt, and pepper, and toss.

*Exchanges/Food Choices: 1 1/2 starch, 2 vegetable, 1 fat*
*Per serving: Calories 150, Calories from Fat 25, Total Fat 2.5 g, Saturated Fat 0 g,*
*Monounsaturated Fat 1.5 g, Cholesterol 0 mg, Sodium 65 mg, Potassium 520 mg,*
*Total Carbohydrate 29 g, Dietary Fiber 5 g, Sugars 7 g, Protein 4 g, Phosphorus 90 mg*

## Shopping List:

3/4 pound boneless, skinless chicken thighs
1 jar reduced-fat mayonnaise
1 bottle prepared horseradish
1 container panko bread crumbs
1/2 pound sweet potatoes
1 package sugar snap peas (6 ounces needed)

## Staples:

Olive oil cooking spray
Salt and black peppercorns
Minced garlic
Olive oil

## Helpful Hint:

■ Boneless, skinless chicken breasts can be used instead of thighs.

# Hot Pepper Chicken with Sweet Pepper Potatoes

*Hot peppers and honey make this a sweet and spicy, quick chicken dinner. Sweet potatoes cooked with fresh red bell peppers make an unusual and surprisingly quick side dish. The potatoes cook in only 5 minutes in a microwave oven.*

## Countdown:

- Prepare ingredients.
- Start sweet potatoes.
- Make chicken.
- Finish sweet potatoes.

### Hot Pepper Chicken

Serves: 2 / Serving Size: 5 ounces chicken, 2 tablespoons sauce

> 3/4 pound boneless, skinless chicken breasts
> 2 tablespoons flour
> 1 teaspoon crushed red pepper
> Salt and freshly ground black pepper, to taste
> 1 tablespoon olive oil
> 2 tablespoons honey
> 2 tablespoons Dijon mustard

1. Place chicken between 2 pieces of plastic wrap or foil. Flatten with a meat mallet or the bottom of a heavy skillet until the breasts are about 1/2 inch thick.

2. In a small bowl, mix the flour, the crushed red pepper, and salt and pepper. Dip flattened chicken breasts in the mixture, making sure all sides are coated.

3. Heat oil in a nonstick skillet over medium-high heat. Sauté chicken for 3 minutes, then turn and cook on second side for 3 minutes. A meat thermometer inserted into chicken should read 165°F.

4. While chicken cooks, mix honey and mustard together. Remove chicken to 2 dinner plates and spread mustard sauce on top.

*Exchanges/Food Choices: 1 starch, 5 lean protein, 1 fat*
*Per serving: Calories 350, Calories from Fat 110, Total Fat 12 g, Saturated Fat 2 g,*
*Monounsaturated Fat 7 g, Cholesterol 125 mg, Sodium 450 mg, Potassium 620 mg,*
*Total Carbohydrate 21 g, Dietary Fiber <1 g, Sugars 17 g, Protein 40 g, Phosphorus 385 mg*

# Sweet Pepper Potatoes

Serves: 2 / Serving Size: 1/2 cup vegetables, 1/2 cup potatoes

> 1/2 pound sweet potatoes, peeled and cut into 1-inch pieces (about
>   1 3/4 cups)
> 1 medium red bell pepper, seeded and cut into 1-inch pieces (about 1 cup)
> 2 teaspoons olive oil
> Salt and freshly ground black pepper, to taste

1. Place sweet potatoes and red bell pepper in a microwave-safe bowl. Cover with plastic wrap or a plate. Microwave on high 5 minutes. Let stand 1 minute.

2. Remove cover and add olive oil and salt and pepper. Toss well and serve with chicken.

*Exchanges/Food Choices: 1 starch, 1 vegetable, 1 fat*
*Per serving: Calories 150, Calories from Fat 40, Total Fat 4.5 g, Saturated Fat 0.5 g,*
*Monounsaturated Fat 3.5 g, Cholesterol 0 mg, Sodium 65 mg, Potassium 480 mg,*
*Total Carbohydrate 26 g, Dietary Fiber 4 g, Sugars 7 g, Protein 2 g, Phosphorus 65 mg*

## Shopping List:

3/4 pound boneless, skinless chicken
   breasts
1 bottle crushed red pepper
1 small bottle honey
1 bottle Dijon mustard
1/2 pound sweet potatoes
1 medium red bell pepper

## Staples:

Flour
Salt and black peppercorns
Olive oil

## Helpful Hints:

- Crushed red pepper, sometimes called hot pepper flakes, can be found in the spice section of the supermarket.
- Green or yellow bell peppers can be substituted for the red bell pepper. Alternatively, canned pimentos can be added to the cooked sweet potatoes.

# Lemon-Pepper Chicken with Carrot and Zucchini Cannellini Beans

*Chicken takes on the spicy, citrus flavor of lemon and cracked black pepper in this hot and refreshing dish. Cannellini beans with carrots and zucchini make a colorful side dish.*

## Countdown:
- Marinate chicken.
- Make side dish.
- Finish chicken.

### Lemon-Pepper Chicken

Serves: 2 / Serving Size: 5 ounces chicken

> 1/4 cup fresh lemon juice
> 1 1/2 tablespoons olive oil
> 1 tablespoon cracked black pepper
> 3/4 pound boneless, skinless chicken breasts

1. Mix lemon juice, olive oil, and pepper together in a small bowl or plastic bag. Remove visible fat from chicken, poke several holes at varying intervals in the chicken, and add chicken to the lemon juice mixture. Let marinate while preparing side dish.

2. Heat a stove-top grill.

3. Remove chicken from marinade, reserving marinade, and sear the chicken on one side for 2 minutes. Turn and sear second side for 2 more minutes. Reduce heat and continue to cook 5–7 minutes. (Chicken can also be cooked under a broiler, cooking for 3–4 minutes per side.)

4. Baste chicken with the reserved marinade as it cooks. A meat thermometer inserted into chicken should read 165°F.

*Exchanges/Food Choices: 5 lean protein, 2 fat*
*Per serving: Calories 310, Calories from Fat 135, Total Fat 15 g, Saturated Fat 2.5 g, Monounsaturated Fat 9 g, Cholesterol 125 mg, Sodium 80 mg, Potassium 650 mg, Total Carbohydrate 4 g, Dietary Fiber 1 g, Sugars <1 g, Protein 39 g, Phosphorus 370 mg*

# Carrot and Zucchini Cannellini Beans

Serves: 2 / Serving Size: 1 cup vegetables, 3/4 cup beans

> 1 cup sliced carrots
> 1 cup sliced zucchini
> 1/2 cup fat-free, low-sodium chicken stock
> 1 1/2 cups low-sodium cannellini beans, rinsed and drained
> 2 teaspoons minced garlic
> Salt and freshly ground black pepper, to taste

1. Add carrots, zucchini, and chicken stock to a medium-size saucepan.

2. Bring to a boil over medium-high heat and cover. Cook 5 minutes.

3. Add the cannellini beans and garlic. Simmer 2–3 minutes to warm the beans. Add salt and pepper to taste, and serve.

*Exchanges/Food Choices: 3 starch, 1 vegetable*
*Per serving: Calories 270, Calories from Fat 10, Total Fat 1 g, Saturated Fat 0 g,*
*Monounsaturated Fat 0 g, Cholesterol 0 mg, Sodium 85 mg, Potassium 1110 mg,*
*Total Carbohydrate 51 g, Dietary Fiber 12 g, Sugars 7 g, Protein 17 g, Phosphorus 350 mg*

## Shopping List:

2 lemons
1 bottle cracked black pepper
3/4 pound boneless, skinless chicken
   breasts
1 package sliced carrots
1 small zucchini
1 can low-sodium cannellini beans

## Staples:

Olive oil
Fat-free, low-sodium chicken stock
Minced garlic
Salt and black peppercorns

## Helpful Hints:

- Cracked black pepper can be found in the spice section of the market.
- Navy beans can be used instead of cannellini beans.

## Shop Smart:

- Look for fat-free, low-sodium chicken stock or broth with 20 calories per cup and about 150 mg sodium per cup.

# Mango Salsa Pan-Roasted Chicken and Hot Peanut Rice

*Chicken with chunky mango salsa makes a sweet and spicy dinner.*
*To cube mango: slice off each side as close to the seed as possible. Take the*
*mango half in your hand, skin side down. Score the fruit in a crisscross pattern*
*through to the skin. Bend the skin backwards so that the cubes pop up. Slice*
*the cubes away from the skin. Score and slice any fruit left on the pit.*

## Countdown:

- Cut mango cubes and make salsa.
- Start rice and make chicken while rice cooks.

## Mango Salsa Pan-Roasted Chicken

Serves: 2 / Serving Size: 5 ounces chicken, 1/2 cup fruit salsa

> 1 cup 1/4-inch mango cubes
> 1 teaspoon sugar
> 2 tablespoons coarsely chopped red onion
> 1 small jalapeño pepper, seeded and chopped (about 1 tablespoon)
> 1 1/2 teaspoons ground cumin, divided
> 1 tablespoon fresh lime juice
> Salt, to taste
> 2 tablespoons chopped fresh cilantro
> 3/4 pound boneless, skinless chicken breasts
> 1 tablespoon olive oil
> Freshly ground black pepper, to taste

1. To make mango salsa, place mango cubes in a medium-size bowl and sprinkle with sugar. Add onion and jalapeño pepper. Mix 1/2 teaspoon cumin and lime juice together, and drizzle over ingredients. Add salt to taste. Toss well and sprinkle with cilantro.

2. Remove all visible fat from chicken. Place between 2 pieces of plastic wrap or foil. Flatten with a meat mallet or the bottom of a heavy skillet to about a 1/2-inch thickness. Sprinkle the remaining 1 teaspoon ground cumin over the chicken.

3. Heat oil in a nonstick skillet over medium-high heat. Cook chicken 3 minutes per side. Add salt and pepper to taste. A meat thermometer should read 165°F.

4. Remove to 2 plates and serve with salsa on top.

*Exchanges/Food Choices: 1 fruit, 5 1/2 lean protein, 1 fat*
*Per serving: Calories 340, Calories from Fat 110, Total Fat 12 g, Saturated Fat 2 g,*
*Monounsaturated Fat 6 g, Cholesterol 125 mg, Sodium 85 mg, Potassium 790 mg,*
*Total Carbohydrate 17 g, Dietary Fiber 2 g, Sugars 14 g, Protein 40 g, Phosphorus 385 mg*

# Hot Peanut Rice

Serves: 2 / Serving Size: 3/4 cup rice

> 1 teaspoon olive oil
> 1/4 cup coarsely chopped red onion
> 1/2 cup long-grain white rice
> 1 cup water
> 2 tablespoons dry-roasted, unsalted peanuts
> 1/4 teaspoon cayenne pepper
> 1 scallion, washed and sliced
> Salt and freshly ground black pepper, to taste

1. Heat oil in a nonstick skillet over medium-high heat, and add onion and rice. Sauté 2 minutes, tossing to coat rice with oil.

2. Add water and bring to a simmer. Cover and continue to simmer 15 minutes until rice is cooked through and liquid is absorbed.

3. Meanwhile, place peanuts in a small bowl and sprinkle with cayenne. When rice is cooked, stir in peanuts and scallion. Add salt and pepper to taste, and serve.

*Exchanges/Food Choices: 2 1/2 starch, 1 1/2 fat*
*Per serving: Calories 250, Calories from Fat 70, Total Fat 7 g, Saturated Fat 1 g,*
*Monounsaturated Fat 4 g, Cholesterol 0 mg, Sodium 5 mg, Potassium 170 mg,*
*Total Carbohydrate 42 g, Dietary Fiber 2 g, Sugars 2 g, Protein 6 g, Phosphorus 95 mg*

## Shopping List:

1 ripe mango
1 small jalapeño pepper
1 bottle ground cumin
1 lime
1 small bunch cilantro
3/4 pound boneless, skinless chicken breasts
1 container dry-roasted, unsalted peanuts
1 bottle cayenne pepper
1 small bunch scallions

## Staples:

Sugar
Red onion
Salt and black peppercorns
Olive oil
Long-grain white rice

## Helpful Hints:

■ Ripe peaches can be substituted for mango.
■ If you like your salsa hot, add more jalapeño pepper.
■ Chopped red onion is used in both recipes. Chop at one time and divide accordingly. Any type of onion can be used.
■ Make sure your bottles of dried spices are less than 6 months old.

# Orange-Honey Chicken with Garlic Zucchini and Grape Tomatoes

*Orange, almonds, and honey flavor chicken cutlets in this quick dinner. Boneless, skinless chicken cutlets, found in most supermarkets, are about 1/2 inch thick. They cook in just 4–5 minutes. A colorful side dish of zucchini strips and grape tomatoes tossed in olive oil and garlic completes the meal.*

## Countdown:

- Prepare ingredients.
- Make zucchini and tomatoes, and set aside.
- Make chicken.

### Orange-Honey Chicken

Serves: 2 / Serving Size: 5 ounces chicken, 5 tablespoons sauce, 1 slice bread

| | |
|---|---|
| 2 tablespoons plus 1 teaspoon cornstarch, divided | 2 teaspoons olive oil |
| Salt and freshly ground black pepper, to taste | 1/2 cup plus 1 tablespoon orange juice, divided |
| 3/4 pound boneless, skinless chicken breast cutlets (1/2 inch thick) | 2 tablespoons honey |
| | 2 tablespoons sliced almonds |
| | 2 slices whole-grain country bread |

1. Mix 2 tablespoons cornstarch and salt and pepper on a plate. Dip chicken cutlets into cornstarch mixture and coat both sides. Shake off excess.

2. Heat oil in a nonstick skillet over medium-high heat. Add the cutlets and sauté 2 minutes. Turn and sauté 2 more minutes. A meat thermometer inserted into chicken should read 165°F.

3. Remove chicken to 2 plates and add 1/2 cup orange juice to the skillet, scraping up the brown bits in the skillet. Add the honey and mix until honey is dissolved. Mix the remaining 1 teaspoon cornstarch and 1 tablespoon orange juice together, and add to the skillet. Stir until the sauce starts to thicken, about 1 minute.

4. Spoon sauce over chicken and sprinkle almonds on top. Serve bread on the side.

*Exchanges/Food Choices: 2 starch, 1 fruit, 5 1/2 lean protein, 1 fat*
*Per serving: Calories 510, Calories from Fat 150, Total Fat 17 g, Saturated Fat 2.5 g, Monounsaturated Fat 9 g, Cholesterol 125 mg, Sodium 180 mg, Potassium 890 mg, Total Carbohydrate 44 g, Dietary Fiber 4 g, Sugars 25 g, Protein 45 g, Phosphorus 500 mg*

# Garlic Zucchini and Grape Tomatoes

Serves: 2 / Serving Size: 1 1/4 cups vegetables

**1/2 pound zucchini (about 2 cups)**
**1 teaspoon minced garlic**
**2 teaspoons olive oil**
**1 cup grape tomatoes**
**Salt and freshly ground black pepper, to taste**

1. Wash zucchini and slice lengthwise into strips.

2. Place in a microwave-safe bowl and add the garlic. Cover with a plate or plastic wrap and microwave on high 2 minutes.

3. Remove and add the olive oil, tomatoes, and salt and pepper. Cover again and let the tomatoes warm in the bowl while you prepare the chicken.

**Stove-top Method:** Heat oil in a nonstick skillet over medium-high heat. Add the garlic and zucchini. Sauté 3 minutes. Add the tomatoes and sauté another 2 minutes. Add salt and pepper to taste.

*Exchanges/Food Choices: 1 vegetable, 1 fat*
*Per serving: Calories 80, Calories from Fat 45, Total Fat 5 g, Saturated Fat 0.5 g,*
*Monounsaturated Fat 3.5 g, Cholesterol 0 mg, Sodium 15 mg, Potassium 520 mg,*
*Total Carbohydrate 8 g, Dietary Fiber 2 g, Sugars 5 g, Protein 2 g, Phosphorus 70 mg*

## Shopping List:

3/4 pound boneless, skinless chicken breast cutlets
1 small container orange juice
1 small bottle honey
1 package sliced almonds
1 loaf whole-grain country bread
1/2 pound zucchini
1 package grape tomatoes

## Staples:

Cornstarch
Salt and black peppercorns
Olive oil
Minced garlic

## Helpful Hints:

- Two crushed garlic cloves can be used instead of minced garlic.
- Boneless, skinless chicken breast can be used instead of cutlets. Flatten to 1/2-inch thickness.

# Oven-Fried Chicken with Creamed Corn and Lima Beans

*Fried chicken is extremely popular, especially the fast-food version. I decided to bake this chicken in the oven and give it a crunchy crust without frying it. Placing the baking tray in the oven to preheat will cook the bottom side of the chicken without having to turn it.*

## Countdown:

- Marinate chicken.
- Prepare all ingredients.
- Coat chicken with cracker crumbs and place in preheated 400°F oven.
- While chicken bakes, prepare creamed corn and lima beans.

## Oven-Fried Chicken

Serves: 2 / Serving Size: 5 ounces chicken

| | |
|---|---|
| 1/2 cup skim milk | 2 teaspoons paprika |
| 1/2 teaspoon cayenne pepper | 1 teaspoon dried thyme |
| 2 6-ounce boneless, skinless chicken breasts | Salt and freshly ground black pepper, to taste |
| 1/4 cup cracker meal | 1 egg white |
| 1/4 cup finely chopped dry-roasted, unsalted peanuts | Olive oil cooking spray |

1. Preheat oven to 400°F. Line a baking tray with foil and place in oven to warm.

2. Mix milk and cayenne pepper together in a bowl.

3. Place the chicken between two sheets of plastic wrap or foil and flatten with a meat mallet or the bottom of a heavy skillet to about 1/2-inch thickness. Add chicken to the milk and marinate while you prepare the other ingredients.

4. Mix cracker meal, peanuts, paprika, thyme, and salt and pepper together. Remove chicken from milk and roll in cracker meal mixture. Dip in egg white and roll again in cracker meal, coating both sides.

5. Remove baking tray from oven and spray with olive oil cooking spray. Place chicken on tray and spray with olive oil cooking spray. Bake 10 minutes or until meat thermometer reaches 165°F when inserted into chicken.

*Exchanges/Food Choices: 1 starch, 6 lean protein, 1 1/2 fat*
*Per serving: Calories 420, Calories from Fat 140, Total Fat 16 g, Saturated Fat 2.5 g, Monounsaturated Fat 7 g, Cholesterol 125 mg, Sodium 125 mg, Potassium 830 mg, Total Carbohydrate 19 g, Dietary Fiber 3 g, Sugars 3 g, Protein 47 g, Phosphorus 480 mg*

# Creamed Corn and Lima Beans

Serves: 2 / Serving Size: 1/2 cup vegetables, 1/2 cup tomato

>    Olive oil cooking spray
>    1/2 cup frozen corn kernels
>    1/2 cup frozen lima beans
>    2 teaspoons canola oil
>    1 tablespoon flour
>    1/2 cup skim milk
>    Salt and freshly ground black pepper, to taste
>    1 medium tomato, sliced

1. Heat a nonstick skillet over medium-high heat. Spray with olive oil cooking spray.

2. Add corn and lima beans. Sauté 2–3 minutes or until vegetables are heated through.

3. Draw vegetables to the sides of the pan, and add oil and flour. Mix to form a paste. Slowly add the milk, stirring to form a creamy sauce.

4. Draw the vegetables into the sauce and mix well. Add salt and pepper to taste. Serve with sliced tomatoes on the side.

*Exchanges/Food Choices: 1 1/2 starch, 1 1/2 fat*
*Per serving: Calories 200, Calories from Fat 60, Total Fat 7 g, Saturated Fat 0.5 g,*
*Monounsaturated Fat 4.5 g, Cholesterol 0 mg, Sodium 55 mg, Potassium 570 mg,*
*Total Carbohydrate 27 g, Dietary Fiber 4 g, Sugars 7 g, Protein 7 g, Phosphorus 155 mg*

## Shopping List:

1 bottle cayenne pepper
2 6-ounce boneless, skinless chicken breasts
1 box cracker meal
1 bottle dry-roasted, unsalted peanuts
1 bottle paprika
1 bottle dried thyme
1 bag frozen corn kernels
1 bag frozen lima beans
1 medium tomato

## Staples:

Skim milk
Salt and black peppercorns
Eggs
Olive oil cooking spray
Canola oil
Flour

## Helpful Hints:

- Bread crumbs can be substituted for cracker crumbs.
- Any type of unsalted, chopped nuts can be used.
- Make sure your bottles of dried herbs and spices are less than 6 months old.

# Pecan-Crusted, Honey-Glazed Chicken with Rosemary-Garlic Cannellini Beans

*Sweet and tangy honey mustard forms a thick glaze over broiled chicken breasts in this 10-minute dinner. Broken pecan pieces add flavor and crunch. Cannellini beans—large, white Italian kidney beans—are a great accent to the chicken.*

## Countdown:
- Preheat broiler.
- Make chicken.
- While chicken broils, make beans.

### Pecan-Crusted, Honey-Glazed Chicken

Serves: 2 / Serving Size: 5 ounces chicken, 1 tablespoon sauce

Vegetable oil cooking spray
3/4 pound boneless, skinless
  chicken breasts
Salt and freshly ground black
  pepper, to taste

2 tablespoons honey
2 tablespoons Dijon mustard
2 tablespoons chopped unsalted
  pecans

1. Preheat broiler. Line a baking tray with foil and spray with vegetable oil cooking spray.

2. Place chicken between 2 pieces of plastic wrap and flatten with the bottom of a heavy pan or meat mallet to about 1/2-inch thickness. Place chicken on foil. Broil 5 inches from heat for 3 minutes. Turn chicken over, add salt and pepper to taste, and broil 3 more minutes. A meat thermometer inserted into chicken should read 165°F.

3. Mix honey and mustard together. Remove chicken from broiler and spoon honey mustard over chicken. Broil 1 additional minute.

4. Remove from broiler and sprinkle pecans over chicken. Divide chicken between 2 dinner plates and pour juices from the baking tray on top of chicken.

*Exchanges/Food Choices: 1 1/2 starch, 1 1/2 fat*
*Per serving: Calories 350, Calories from Fat 110, Total Fat 12 g, Saturated Fat 1.5 g, Monounsaturated Fat 6 g, Cholesterol 125 mg, Sodium 460 mg, Potassium 630 mg, Total Carbohydrate 20 g, Dietary Fiber 1 g, Sugars 18 g, Protein 40 g, Phosphorus 395 mg*

## Rosemary-Garlic Cannellini Beans

Serves: 2 / Serving Size: 1/2 cup

> 1 cup low-sodium canned cannellini beans, rinsed and drained
> 1/4 cup fat-free, low-sodium chicken stock
> 2 garlic cloves, crushed
> 2 teaspoons dried rosemary
> Salt and freshly ground black pepper, to taste

1. Place beans in saucepan with chicken stock, crushed garlic, and rosemary. Simmer 3 minutes to warm through. Add salt and pepper to taste.

**Microwave Method:** Place all ingredients in a microwave-safe bowl and microwave on high 2 minutes. Stir well.

*Exchanges/Food Choices: 2 starch*
*Per serving: Calories 170, Calories from Fat 10, Total Fat 1 g, Saturated Fat 0 g,*
*Monounsaturated Fat 0 g, Cholesterol 0 mg, Sodium 25 mg, Potassium 540 mg,*
*Total Carbohydrate 31 g, Dietary Fiber 8 g, Sugars 2 g, Protein 11 g, Phosphorus 200 mg*

## Shopping List:

3/4 pound boneless, skinless chicken breasts
1 small bottle honey
1 bottle Dijon mustard
1 package unsalted pecans
1 can low-sodium cannellini beans
1 bottle dried rosemary

## Staples:

Vegetable oil cooking spray
Salt and black peppercorns
Fat-free, low-sodium chicken stock
Garlic

## Helpful Hints:

- White navy beans or black beans can be substituted for cannellini beans.
- Make sure your bottles of dried herbs and spices are less than 6 months old.

## Shop Smart:

- Look for fat-free, low-sodium chicken stock or broth with 20 calories per cup and about 150 mg sodium per cup.

# Sangria-Braised Pulled Chicken Sliders with Quick Slaw

*These sliders are made with plump chicken thighs that are cooked in red wine and flavored with cinnamon, star anise, and oranges. Star anise can be found in the spice section of the supermarket. It is a small, star-shaped spice that has a licorice or anise flavor. You can use it in many other dishes. Add a couple to the saucepan when cooking rice or add it to a stir-fry sauce.*

## Countdown:

- Start braised chicken.
- While chicken cooks, make slaw.

### Sangria-Braised Pulled Chicken Sliders

Serves: 2 / Serving Size: 5 ounces chicken, 2 (1-ounce) rolls

| | |
|---|---|
| 3/4 pound boneless, skinless chicken thighs | 1 cinnamon stick |
| 1 teaspoon canola oil | 1 star anise |
| 1 cup sliced carrots | 1 orange cut into wedges |
| 1 cup frozen diced onion, defrosted | 1 cup red wine |
| | 1 tablespoon sugar |
| | 4 mini slider rolls |

1. Remove visible fat from chicken.
2. Heat oil in a medium-size nonstick saucepan over medium-high heat. Add the chicken and brown 2 minutes. Turn and brown 2 more minutes.
3. Add the carrots, onion, cinnamon stick, star anise, orange wedges, red wine, and sugar. Bring to a simmer. Cover and simmer 15 minutes.
4. Remove the chicken with a slotted spoon from the skillet to a plate. A meat thermometer inserted into chicken should read 165°F. Place the liquid in a colander over a bowl and let strain while finishing the chicken. Using 2 forks, shred the chicken.
5. Divide chicken among the 4 sliders. Press the liquid from the vegetables and orange in the colander. Discard orange and vegetables, and spoon the reserved liquid over the chicken in the sliders.

*Exchanges/Food Choices: 2 starch, 2 vegetable, 6 lean protein, 1 fat*
*Per serving: Calories 530, Calories from Fat 110, Total Fat 12 g, Saturated Fat 2.5 g,*
*Monounsaturated Fat 4.5 g, Cholesterol 160 mg, Sodium 490 mg, Potassium 790 mg,*
*Total Carbohydrate 41 g, Dietary Fiber 5 g, Sugars 11 g, Protein 42 g, Phosphorus 495 mg*

## Quick Slaw

Serves: 2 / Serving Size: 3/4 cup

1 1/2 tablespoons reduced-fat mayonnaise
2 tablespoons warm water
1 tablespoon cider vinegar
1/4 cup frozen diced onion, defrosted
1 1/2 cups shredded cabbage
Salt and freshly ground black pepper, to taste

1. Add the reduced-fat mayonnaise, warm water, and cider vinegar to a medium-size bowl. Mix until smooth.
2. Add the onion and shredded cabbage. Mix well. Add salt and pepper to taste, and toss again.

*Exchanges/Food Choices: 1 vegetable, 1 fat*
*Per serving: Calories 60, Calories from Fat 30, Total Fat 3.5 g, Saturated Fat 0.5 g,*
*Monounsaturated Fat 1 g, Cholesterol 0 mg, Sodium 95 mg, Potassium 125 mg,*
*Total Carbohydrate 5 g, Dietary Fiber 2 g, Sugars 3 g, Protein <1 g, Phosphorus 20 mg*

## Shopping List:

3/4 pound boneless, skinless chicken thighs
1 package frozen diced onion
1 container cinnamon sticks
1 package star anise
1 orange
1 small bottle red wine
1 package mini slider rolls
1 bottle reduced-fat mayonnaise
1 bottle cider vinegar
1 package shredded cabbage

## Staples:

Canola oil
Carrots
Sugar
Salt and black peppercorns

## Helpful Hints:

- Use one hamburger roll per person if slider rolls aren't available.
- Two teaspoons of five-spice powder can be used instead of star anise. Or you can omit the star anise. The dish will taste different, but it will still be delicious.
- Find sliced carrots and shredded cabbage in the produce section of the market.
- A quick way to defrost frozen onion is to place it in a sieve under hot tap water. Squeeze out extra liquid. Defrost onion for both recipes at one time. Divide according to recipes.

# Savory Sage Chicken with Zucchini and Tomato Rice

*Chicken dusted with a sage coating is flavored with a vermouth sauce
in this quick dinner. The vermouth adds flavor without fuss.*

## Countdown:

- Prepare all ingredients.
- Start rice.
- Make chicken.
- Complete rice.

## Savory Sage Chicken

Serves: 2 / Serving Size: 5 ounces chicken, 2 tablespoons sauce

> **3/4 pound boneless, skinless chicken breasts**
> **2 tablespoons flour**
> **3 teaspoons ground sage**
> **Salt and freshly ground black pepper, to taste**
> **3 teaspoons olive oil**
> **1/4 cup dry vermouth**
> **1/4 cup water**

1. Remove visible fat from chicken.

2. Mix together flour, sage, and salt and pepper. Roll chicken in mixture, pressing flour into chicken on both sides. Shake off excess flour.

3. Heat oil in a nonstick skillet over medium-high heat. Add chicken to skillet and cook 5 minutes, turn over, and cook 5 more minutes. A meat thermometer inserted into chicken should read 165°F.

4. Remove chicken to a plate and raise heat under skillet to high. Add vermouth and water, and reduce for 2–3 minutes. Pour the sauce over the chicken.

*Exchanges/Food Choices: 5 lean protein, 1 1/2 fat*
*Per serving: Calories 300, Calories from Fat 100, Total Fat 11 g, Saturated Fat 2 g,*
*Monounsaturated Fat 6 g, Cholesterol 125 mg, Sodium 80 mg, Potassium 580 mg,*
*Total Carbohydrate 3 g, Dietary Fiber 0 g, Sugars 0 g, Protein 39 g, Phosphorus 365 mg*

# Zucchini and Tomato Rice

Serves: 2 / Serving Size: 3/4 cup rice, 1 cup vegetables

**1/2 cup long-grain white rice**
**1/2 pound zucchini, sliced (large-diameter slices cut in half)**
**1 medium tomato, cut into 2-inch cubes**
**1 teaspoon olive oil**
**2 tablespoons shredded, part-skim mozzarella cheese**
**Salt and freshly ground black pepper, to taste**

1. Bring a large saucepan with 2–3 quarts water to a boil.

2. Add the rice and boil 5 minutes. Add the zucchini and continue to boil 5 minutes. Drain, and return rice and zucchini to the pan.

3. Add the tomato, olive oil, mozzarella cheese, and salt and pepper. Toss well and serve.

*Exchanges/Food Choices: 2 starch, 2 vegetable, 1 fat*
*Per serving: Calories 250, Calories from Fat 40, Total Fat 4.5 g, Saturated Fat 1.5 g,*
*Monounsaturated Fat 2 g, Cholesterol 5 mg, Sodium 75 mg, Potassium 570 mg,*
*Total Carbohydrate 44 g, Dietary Fiber 3 g, Sugars 5 g, Protein 8 g, Phosphorus 160 mg*

## Shopping List:

3/4 pound boneless, skinless chicken breasts
1 bottle ground sage
1 bottle dry vermouth
1/2 pound zucchini
1 medium tomato
1 small package shredded, part-skim mozzarella cheese

## Staples:

Flour
Salt and black peppercorns
Olive oil
Long-grain white rice

## Helpful Hints:

■ White wine can be substituted for vermouth.
■ Make sure your bottles of dried herbs and spices are less than 6 months old.

# Southwestern Chicken Burgers with Tortilla Salad

*Spicy tomato salsa gives these light, juicy chicken burgers a hint of the Southwest. Look for ground chicken made from chicken breast meat only. If the label just says "ground chicken," then skin, fat, and dark meat may have been added.*

## Countdown:

- Make salad and set aside.
- Prepare chicken burgers.

### Southwestern Chicken Burgers

Serves: 2 / Serving Size: 5 ounces chicken, 2 teaspoons sauce, 1 roll

> 3/4 pound ground, white-meat-only chicken
> 1/4 cup no-sugar-added tomato salsa, drained
> Salt and freshly ground black pepper, to taste
> Olive oil cooking spray
> 2 whole-wheat or whole-grain hamburger rolls (1 1/2 ounces each)
> 1 medium tomato, sliced
> 2 lettuce leaves from the salad side dish
> 1 1/2 tablespoons mayonnaise

1. Mix chicken, salsa, and salt and black pepper together in a small bowl. Shape into burgers about 4 inches round and 1/4–1/2 inch thick.

2. Heat a nonstick skillet over medium-high heat. Spray with olive oil cooking spray and sauté burgers 5 minutes on each side. A meat thermometer inserted into chicken should read 165°F.

3. Meanwhile, spray hamburger rolls with olive oil cooking spray and toast in toaster oven or under broiler.

4. Place cooked chicken burgers on bottom half of each roll. Place 1 tomato slice and a lettuce leaf on top of each burger. Garnish the plate with extra slices of tomato. Spread mayonnaise on the top half of the bun and close the burger.

*Exchanges/Food Choices: 2 starch, 6 lean protein, 1/2 fat*
*Per serving: Calories 450, Calories from Fat 140, Total Fat 16 g, Saturated Fat 2.5 g, Monounsaturated Fat 4.5 g, Cholesterol 130 mg, Sodium 510 mg, Potassium 1020 mg, Total Carbohydrate 27 g, Dietary Fiber 5 g, Sugars 6 g, Protein 46 g, Phosphorus 500 mg*

## Tortilla Salad

Serves: 2 / Serving Size: 2 cups vegetables, 1 tablespoon dressing, 1/4 cup chips

> **4 cups washed, ready-to-eat salad**
> **2 tablespoons reduced-fat oil and vinegar dressing**
> **1/2 cup baked, low-fat tortilla chips**

1. Place salad in bowl and toss with dressing. Sprinkle tortilla chips on top.

*Exchanges/Food Choices: 1/2 starch, 1 vegetable, 1/2 fat*
*Per serving: Calories 90, Calories from Fat 20, Total Fat 2 g, Saturated Fat 0 g,*
*Monounsaturated Fat 0.5 g, Cholesterol 0 mg, Sodium 85 mg, Potassium 280 mg,*
*Total Carbohydrate 15 g, Dietary Fiber 3 g, Sugars 2 g, Protein 3 g, Phosphorus 75 mg*

## Shopping List:

3/4 pound ground, white-meat-only chicken

1 bottle no-sugar-added tomato salsa

1 package whole-wheat or whole-grain hamburger rolls

1 medium tomato

1 bag washed, ready-to-eat salad

1 bag baked, low-fat tortilla chips

## Staples:

Salt and black peppercorns

Olive oil cooking spray

Mayonnaise

Reduced-fat oil and vinegar dressing

## Helpful Hints:

■ Be sure to drain the salsa to keep the hamburgers from being too wet. This will allow them to retain their shape.

■ Any type of washed, ready-to-eat greens can be used.

# Stout-Soused Chicken with Potatoes and Leeks

*Chicken, potatoes, and leeks lightly coated in a stout (a dark, strong beer) and mustard sauce blend perfectly for this meal. Stout is brewed from hops and roasted malt or roasted barley. It has a distinct toasted flavor, which is a favorite of the Irish.*

## Countdown:

- Prepare all ingredients.
- Make dish.

### Stout-Soused Chicken with Potatoes and Leeks

Serves: 2 / Serving Size: 5 ounces chicken, 3/4 cup potatoes, 3/4 cup vegetables, 2 tablespoons sauce

> 1 tablespoon canola oil
> 3/4 pound boneless, skinless chicken thighs
> Salt and freshly ground black pepper, to taste
> 2 medium leeks, cleaned and sliced (about 2 cups)
> 3/4 pound red or yellow potatoes, with skin, cut into 1-inch cubes (about 2 1/2 cups)
> 1/2 cup sliced carrots
> 3/4 cup stout
> 2 cups water
> 2 tablespoons cider vinegar
> 2 tablespoons honey
> 1 1/2 tablespoons coarse-ground mustard
> 1 cup frozen peas
> 3 scallions, sliced (about 1/2 cup)

1. Heat the oil in a nonstick skillet over medium-high heat.

2. Brown chicken 2 minutes, turn over, and brown 2 more minutes. Sprinkle with salt and pepper. Remove to a plate and set aside.

3. Add leeks, potatoes, carrots, stout, water, and cider vinegar to the skillet. Reduce heat to medium. Cover with a lid and simmer 10 minutes or until potatoes are cooked.

4. Mix the honey and mustard together, add to the skillet, and stir well to blend.

5. Return chicken to the skillet, and add the peas. Simmer 3–4 minutes or until chicken is cooked through. A meat thermometer inserted into chicken should read 170°F. Add salt and pepper to taste.

6. Remove chicken and vegetables with a slotted spoon to 2 dishes. Raise heat under skillet and reduce the sauce by half for 1–2 minutes. Spoon sauce over chicken and vegetables, and sprinkle the scallions on top.

*Exchanges/Food Choices: 3 starch, 1 other carbohydrate, 5 lean protein, 1/2 fat*
*Per serving: Calories 560, Calories from Fat 140, Total Fat 15 g, Saturated Fat 2.5 g,*
*Monounsaturated Fat 7 g, Cholesterol 160 mg, Sodium 530 mg, Potassium 1670 mg,*
*Total Carbohydrate 59 g, Dietary Fiber 9 g, Sugars 21 g, Protein 42 g, Phosphorus 515 mg*

## Shopping List:

3/4 pound boneless, skinless chicken thighs
2 medium leeks
3/4 pound red or yellow potatoes
1 package sliced carrots
1 bottle stout
1 bottle cider vinegar
1 small bottle honey
1 jar coarse-ground mustard
1 package frozen peas
1 bunch scallions

## Staples:

Canola oil
Salt and black peppercorns

## Helpful Hints:

■ Dijon mustard can be used instead of coarse-grain mustard.
■ Any type of beer can be used.

# Sweet and Sour Meatballs with Egg Noodles and Peas

*Meatballs in a tangy, sweet tomato sauce is a 1950s comfort food that is back in style. Meatballs freeze well. Make extra for another quick dinner. Look for ground chicken made from chicken breast meat only. If the label just says "ground chicken," then skin, fat, and dark meat may have been added.*

## Countdown:

- Place water for noodles on to boil.
- Make meatballs.
- Make noodles.

### Sweet and Sour Meatballs

Serves: 2 / Serving Size: 5 ounces chicken, 1/2 cup sauce

| | |
|---|---|
| 3/4 pound ground, white-meat-only chicken | 1/2 cup frozen diced onion, defrosted |
| 2 tablespoons bread crumbs | 1 cup low-sodium tomato sauce |
| Salt and freshly ground black pepper, to taste | 1 1/2 tablespoons fresh lemon juice |
| 1 egg white | Sugar substitute equivalent to 4 teaspoons sugar |
| Olive oil cooking spray | 2 tablespoons raisins |

1. Mix ground chicken with bread crumbs, salt and pepper, and egg white. Form into meatballs about 1 1/2 inches in diameter (about 14 balls).

2. Heat a medium-size nonstick skillet, just large enough to hold the meatballs in one layer, over medium-high heat. Spray with olive oil cooking spray. Brown meatballs on all sides, about 5 minutes.

3. While meatballs brown, add onion. Stir onion so that it cooks without browning. Add tomato sauce, lemon juice, sugar substitute, and raisins. Gently simmer 10 minutes, turning balls in sauce once or twice. Add salt and pepper to taste.

4. Taste for a blend of sweet and sour flavors. Add more lemon juice if necessary. Serve over noodles.

*Exchanges/Food Choices: 1 other carbohydrate, 2 vegetable, 5 lean protein*
*Per serving: Calories 340, Calories from Fat 60, Total Fat 7 g, Saturated Fat 1 g,*
*Monounsaturated Fat 2.5 g, Cholesterol 125 mg, Sodium 180 mg, Potassium 1150 mg,*
*Total Carbohydrate 25 g, Dietary Fiber 3 g, Sugars 14 g, Protein 43 g, Phosphorus 425 mg*

## Egg Noodles and Peas

Serves: 2 / Serving Size: 3/4 cup noodles, 1/4 cup vegetables

3 ounces egg noodles (about 2 cups)
1/2 cup frozen peas
1/4 cup water (reserved from cooking noodles)
1 tablespoon olive oil
Salt and freshly ground black pepper, to taste

1. Bring a large pot of water to a boil.

2. Add the noodles. Boil 8 minutes.

3. Add peas and continue to boil 2 minutes.

4. Remove 1/4 cup cooking water to a mixing bowl and add the oil to the bowl.

5. Drain noodles and peas, and add to the bowl. Toss well. Add salt and pepper to taste.

*Exchanges/Food Choices: 2 starch, 1 1/2 fat*
*Per serving: Calories 240, Calories from Fat 80, Total Fat 9 g, Saturated Fat 1.5 g,*
*Monounsaturated Fat 6 g, Cholesterol 35 mg, Sodium 10 mg, Potassium 170 mg,*
*Total Carbohydrate 33 g, Dietary Fiber 3 g, Sugars 3 g, Protein 7 g, Phosphorus 120 mg*

## Shopping List:      Staples:

| Shopping List: | Staples: |
|---|---|
| 3/4 pound ground, white-meat-only chicken | Salt and black peppercorns |
| 1 container bread crumbs | Eggs |
| 1 package frozen diced onion | Olive oil cooking spray |
| 1 can low-sodium tomato sauce | Sugar substitute |
| 1 lemon | Olive oil |
| 1 container raisins | |
| 1 package egg noodles | |
| 1 package frozen peas | |

## Helpful Hints:

- Mix the chicken ingredients with a fork. Wet your hands to help form the meatballs.
- A quick way to defrost the onion is to place it in a sieve and run hot tap water over it. Squeeze out extra liquid.

## Shop Smart:

- Look for low-sodium tomato sauce with 70 calories, 0.5 g fat, and 27 mg sodium per cup.

# Walnut-Crusted Chicken with Tomato and Bean Salad

*Walnuts form a crunchy coating that contrasts with the juicy chicken in this meal. Hot pepper jelly lends a surprise punch. For the salad, just toss ripe tomatoes cut into cubes with rinsed, canned Great Northern beans and Italian dressing.*

## Countdown:

- Make salad and set aside.
- Make chicken.

## Walnut-Crusted Chicken

Serves: 2 / Serving Size: 5 ounces chicken, 2 tablespoons sauce

> **Olive oil cooking spray**
> **3/4 pound boneless, skinless chicken breasts**
> **2 tablespoons hot pepper jam or jelly**
> **2 tablespoons finely chopped walnuts**
> **Salt and freshly ground black pepper, to taste**

1. Heat a nonstick skillet over medium-high heat and spray with olive oil cooking spray.

2. Add chicken and cook 5 minutes. Turn chicken and spread the hot pepper jelly over the cooked side. Press the walnuts into the chicken.

3. Continue to sauté the chicken for 5 more minutes. A meat thermometer inserted into chicken should read 165°F. Sprinkle with salt and pepper to taste, and serve.

*Exchanges/Food Choices: 1 other carbohydrate, 5 lean protein, 1/2 fat*
*Per serving: Calories 330, Calories from Fat 100, Total Fat 11 g, Saturated Fat 1.5 g,*
*Monounsaturated Fat 3 g, Cholesterol 125 mg, Sodium 85 mg, Potassium 610 mg,*
*Total Carbohydrate 16 g, Dietary Fiber <1 g, Sugars 11 g, Protein 39 g, Phosphorus 385 mg*

## Tomato and Bean Salad

Serves: 2 / Serving Size: 1 1/2 cups salad, 1 tablespoon dressing

>  2 medium tomatoes, cut into large cubes (about 2 cups)
>  1 cup small, canned Great Northern beans, drained and rinsed
>  2 tablespoons reduced-fat Italian salad dressing
>  Salt and freshly ground black pepper, to taste
>  2 tablespoons chopped parsley (optional)

1. Place tomatoes and beans in a bowl, and add dressing. Toss well. Add salt and pepper to taste, and mix again. Sprinkle parsley on top (optional).

*Exchanges/Food Choices: 2 starch, 1 vegetable*
*Per serving: Calories 190, Calories from Fat 20, Total Fat 2 g, Saturated Fat 0 g,*
*Monounsaturated Fat 0 g, Cholesterol 0 mg, Sodium 20 mg, Potassium 920 mg,*
*Total Carbohydrate 36 g, Dietary Fiber 9 g, Sugars 7 g, Protein 11 g, Phosphorus 225 mg*

## Shopping List:

3/4 pound boneless, skinless chicken breasts
1 jar hot pepper jam or jelly
1 small package walnut pieces
2 medium tomatoes
1 can small Great Northern beans
1 small bunch parsley (optional)

## Staples:

Olive oil cooking spray
Salt and black peppercorns
Reduced-fat Italian salad dressing

## Helpful Hints:

- Chop the nuts in a food processor.
- Any type of hot pepper jam or jelly can be used.
- Any type of canned beans can be used for the salad.

# Latin and Caribbean

# Brazilian-Style Chicken and Quinoa

*Cumin, cayenne pepper, and coconut milk are among the diverse flavors used in Brazilian dishes. They are featured in this Brazilian sautéed chicken dish served over quinoa. Quinoa is an ancient grain indigenous to the Andes Mountains in South America. It has a nutty flavor, is high in protein, and is a good source of fiber. It's also gluten-free.*

## Countdown:

- Start chicken.
- While chicken cooks, make quinoa.

### Brazilian-Style Chicken

Serves: 2 / Serving Size: 5 ounces chicken, 3/4 cup vegetables

2 chicken breasts, bone in and wings removed (about 3/4 pound each)
2 teaspoons ground cumin
1/4 teaspoon cayenne pepper
1 teaspoon canola oil
1 cup frozen diced onion
1/2 cup fat-free, low-sodium chicken stock
2 cups frozen sliced okra
1/4 cup light coconut milk
Salt and freshly ground black pepper, to taste
1 1/2 tablespoons dry-roasted, unsalted peanuts

1. Remove skin from chicken. Mix cumin and cayenne pepper together and rub over chicken.

2. Heat oil in a medium-size nonstick skillet over medium-high heat. Brown chicken, turning to brown all sides, for 5 minutes.

3. Add the onion, chicken stock, and okra. Bring to a simmer. Reduce heat to medium-low, cover with a lid, and simmer 15 minutes. A meat thermometer inserted into chicken should read 165°F.

4. Add coconut milk and salt and pepper, and mix into sauce. Sprinkle peanuts on top. Serve over quinoa.

*Exchanges/Food Choices: 1/2 other carbohydrate, 2 vegetable, 6 lean protein*
*Per serving: Calories 350, Calories from Fat 120, Total Fat 13 g, Saturated Fat 3 g, Monounsaturated Fat 4.5 g, Cholesterol 125 mg, Sodium 140 mg, Potassium 1130 mg, Total Carbohydrate 17 g, Dietary Fiber 6 g, Sugars 5 g, Protein 45 g, Phosphorus 505 mg*

## Quinoa

Serves: 2 / Serving Size: 3/4 cup

**1/2 cup quinoa**
**1 1/2 cups water**
**Salt and freshly ground black pepper, to taste**

1. Place quinoa in a colander or sieve with small openings and run cold water over the grains.
2. Place the quinoa and water in a saucepan. Bring to a boil over high heat. Reduce heat to medium, cover with a lid, and cook 10 minutes. All of the water should be absorbed. If the pan runs dry before the quinoa is cooked, add more water.
3. Add salt and pepper to taste. Place quinoa on a plate, and serve chicken and sauce on top.

*Exchanges/Food Choices: 2 starch*
*Per serving: Calories 160, Calories from Fat 25, Total Fat 2.5 g, Saturated Fat 0 g,*
*Monounsaturated Fat 0.5 g, Cholesterol 0 mg, Sodium 0 mg, Potassium 240 mg,*
*Total Carbohydrate 27 g, Dietary Fiber 3 g, Sugars 0 g, Protein 6 g, Phosphorus 195 mg*

## Shopping List:

2 chicken breasts, bone in and wings removed (about 3/4 pound each)
1 bottle ground cumin
1 bottle cayenne pepper
1 package frozen diced onion
1 package frozen sliced okra
1 can light coconut milk
1 container dry-roasted, unsalted peanuts
1 package quinoa

## Staples:

Canola oil
Fat-free, low-sodium chicken stock
Salt and black peppercorns

## Helpful Hints:

- Green beans can be substituted for okra. Add them to the chicken after it has simmered for 10 minutes.
- Canned coconut milk can be found in the ethnic section of the market.
- Make sure your bottles of dried herbs and spices are less than 6 months old.

## Shop Smart:

- Look for fat-free, low-sodium chicken stock or broth with 20 calories per cup and about 150 mg sodium per cup.
- Look for light coconut milk with 150 calories, 12 g fat, and 45 mg sodium per cup.

# Chicken-Mushroom Quesadillas with Corn and Black Bean Salad

*These Tex-Mex sandwiches are pan-fried and served with a quick Corn and Black Bean Salad. A variety of textures and flavors—from the earthy, meaty mushrooms to the soft cheese and crisp tortillas—combine to create this tasty, satisfying meal.*

## Countdown:

- Make salad and set aside.
- Make quesadillas.

### Chicken-Mushroom Quesadillas

Serves: 2 / Serving Size: 3 ounces chicken, 3/4 cup vegetables, 1 tortilla, 1 tablespoon cheese

> 1/2 pound boneless, skinless chicken breast cutlets (1/2 inch thick)
> 1/2 teaspoon ground cumin
> Olive oil cooking spray
> 1/4 pound sliced, baby bello mushrooms (about 1 2/3 cups)
> 2 cups washed, ready-to-eat spinach
> Salt and freshly ground black pepper, to taste
> 2 8-inch flour tortillas (1 ounce each)
> 1/4 cup shredded, reduced-fat cheddar cheese, divided

1. Sprinkle chicken with ground cumin, covering all sides.

2. Heat a nonstick skillet over medium-high heat and spray with olive oil cooking spray. Add the chicken and mushrooms, and sauté 3–4 minutes or until mushrooms are soft and chicken cooked. A meat thermometer inserted into chicken should read 165°F.

3. Stir in spinach for about 1 minute until it wilts. Add salt and pepper to taste. Remove chicken and vegetables to a bowl.

4. Using the same skillet, spray again with olive oil cooking spray and add one tortilla. Heat about 1 minute or until the bottom is golden. Turn tortilla over

---

*Exchanges/Food Choices: 1 starch, 1 vegetable, 4 1/2 lean protein*
*Per serving: Calories 300, Calories from Fat 100, Total Fat 11 g, Saturated Fat 2 g,*
*Monounsaturated Fat 5 g, Cholesterol 85 mg, Sodium 460 mg, Potassium 790 mg,*
*Total Carbohydrate 21 g, Dietary Fiber 7 g, Sugars 2 g, Protein 36 g, Phosphorus 425 mg*

and spread half the chicken mixture over half the tortilla. Sprinkle half the shredded cheese over the chicken. Gently fold tortilla in half, cover skillet with a lid, and sauté 1 minute.

5. Remove to a dinner plate and repeat step 4 for second tortilla.

## Corn and Black Bean Salad

Serves: 2 / Serving Size: 1 cup vegetables, 1 tablespoon dressing

> 1 cup frozen corn kernels, defrosted
> 1 cup reduced-sodium, canned black beans, drained and rinsed
> 2 tablespoons reduced-fat oil and vinegar dressing
> Salt and freshly ground black pepper, to taste

1. Place corn and black beans in a bowl. Add dressing and salt and pepper to taste. Toss well.

*Exchanges/Food Choices: 2 starch, 1/2 fat*
*Per serving: Calories 180, Calories from Fat 20, Total Fat 2 g, Saturated Fat 0 g,*
*Monounsaturated Fat 0.5 g, Cholesterol 0 mg, Sodium 105 mg, Potassium 530 mg,*
*Total Carbohydrate 35 g, Dietary Fiber 10 g, Sugars 3 g, Protein 9 g, Phosphorus 180 mg*

## Shopping List:

1/2 pound boneless, skinless chicken breast cutlets
1 bottle ground cumin
1/4 pound sliced, baby bello mushrooms
1 bag washed, ready-to-eat spinach
1 package 8-inch flour tortillas
1 package shredded, reduced-fat cheddar cheese
1 package frozen corn kernels
1 can reduced-sodium black beans

## Staples:

Olive oil cooking spray
Salt and black peppercorns
Reduced-fat oil and vinegar dressing

## Helpful Hints:

■ A quick way to defrost corn kernels is to place them in a strainer in the sink and run hot water through them. Squeeze out extra liquid.

■ If you prefer, you can use 2 skillets and make both quesadillas at the same time.

■ Make sure your bottles of dried herbs and spices are less than 6 months old.

## Shop Smart:

■ Look for light tortillas, 8–9 inches in diameter, weighing 39 g (or 1 1/2 ounces), with 80 calories, 2 g fat, and 250 mg sodium per tortilla.

# Chicken Enchiladas with Esquites

*This enchilada is filled with chicken and refried beans and topped with a spicy tomato sauce. Esquites, or fried corn, is a typical Mexican side dish.*

## Countdown:

- Prepare enchiladas.
- Sauté esquites.
- Heat enchiladas in microwave oven.

## Chicken Enchiladas

Serves: 2 / Serving Size: 3 ounces chicken, 3 tablespoons sauce, 2 tortillas, 1 tablespoon cheese

> 2 teaspoons canola oil
> 1/2 pound boneless, skinless chicken breast cutlets (1/2 inch thick)
> Salt and freshly ground black pepper, to taste
> 4 6-inch corn tortillas
> 1/2 cup canned, fat-free refried beans
> 1 cup chopped fresh cilantro
> 1 cup low-sodium tomato sauce
> 1/8 teaspoon hot pepper sauce
> 1/4 cup shredded, reduced-fat mexican-style cheese

1. Heat canola oil in a nonstick skillet over medium-high heat.
2. Cut chicken into 1/4-inch-thick strips and add to the skillet. Season with salt and pepper to taste. Sauté 2 minutes, making sure all sides are cooked.
3. Place tortillas on a countertop. Divide chicken evenly among the 4 tortillas. Spread refried beans over the chicken and sprinkle cilantro on top. Roll up tortillas and place, seam side down, in a microwave-safe dish just big enough to hold them.
4. Mix tomato sauce and hot pepper sauce together, and spoon over tortillas. Cover with another dish or plastic wrap and microwave on high for 2 minutes. Remove cover and sprinkle with cheese.
5. Cover and microwave 1 minute. Divide between 2 plates.

**Oven Method:** Enchiladas can be placed in an oven preheated to 400°F for 10 minutes to warm through or under a broiler for 5 minutes.

*Exchanges/Food Choices: 2 1/2 starch, 1 vegetable, 4 1/2 lean protein*
*Per serving: Calories 420, Calories from Fat 110, Total Fat 12 g, Saturated Fat 3 g,*
*Monounsaturated Fat 5 g, Cholesterol 95 mg, Sodium 460 mg, Potassium 1240 mg,*
*Total Carbohydrate 42 g, Dietary Fiber 8 g, Sugars 6 g, Protein 37 g, Phosphorus 600 mg*

## Esquites

Serves: 2 / Serving Size: 1 cup

> 2 teaspoons canola oil
> 1 cup frozen diced onion, defrosted
> 1 cup frozen diced green bell pepper, defrosted
> 3/4 cup frozen corn kernels, defrosted
> Several drops hot pepper sauce
> Salt and freshly ground black pepper, to taste

1. In the nonstick skillet used for the chicken, heat oil over medium-high heat. Add onion, green peppers, and corn. Sauté 5 minutes. Add hot pepper sauce, and salt and pepper to taste.

*Exchanges/Food Choices: 1 starch, 1 fat*
*Per serving: Calories 120, Calories from Fat 45, Total Fat 5 g, Saturated Fat 0 g,*
*Monounsaturated Fat 3 g, Cholesterol 0 mg, Sodium 20 mg, Potassium 290 mg,*
*Total Carbohydrate 18 g, Dietary Fiber 3 g, Sugars 5 g, Protein 3 g, Phosphorus 60 mg*

## Shopping List:

1/2 pound boneless, skinless chicken breast cutlets
1 package 6-inch corn tortillas
1 can fat-free refried beans
1 bunch cilantro
1 small bottle/can low-sodium tomato sauce
1 package shredded, reduced-fat mexican-style cheese
1 package frozen diced onion
1 package frozen diced green bell pepper
1 package frozen corn kernels

## Staples:

Canola oil
Salt and black peppercorns
Hot pepper sauce

## Helpful Hints:

- Shredded monterey jack can be used instead of mexican-style cheese
- A quick way to defrost the onion, green peppers, and corn is to place them in a sieve and run hot tap water over them. Squeeze out extra liquid.

## Shop Smart:

- Look for corn tortillas, 6 inches in diameter, weighing 26 g (a little under 1 ounce), with 58 calories, 7 g fat, and 3 mg sodium per tortilla.
- Look for canned fat-free refried beans with 182 calories, 1 g fat, and 1012 mg sodium per cup.
- Look for low-sodium tomato sauce with 70 calories, 0.5 g fat, and 27 mg sodium per cup.

# Chimichurri Chicken with Red Pepper and Tomato Penne

*Chimichurri sauce over sautéed chicken is a Latin favorite. Parsley, garlic, hot red pepper, oil, and vinegar are the basic ingredients for this piquant sauce that is used throughout South America. Bottled low-sodium chimichurri sauce can be used instead of preparing your own.*

## Countdown:

- Place water for pasta on to boil.
- Make chimichurri sauce.
- Cook pasta.
- Cook chicken and sauce.
- Finish pasta dish.

## Chimichurri Chicken

Serves: 2 / Serving Size: 5 ounces chicken, 2 tablespoons sauce

| | |
|---|---|
| 1 garlic clove, crushed | 2 teaspoons cider vinegar |
| 1 1/2 cups fresh parsley leaves | 3/4 pound boneless, skinless |
| Pinch red pepper flakes | chicken breasts |
| 1/4 cup water | Salt and freshly ground |
| 4 teaspoons olive oil, divided | black pepper, to taste |

1. To crush garlic, add it to the food processor through the feed tube with the blades running. Again with the motor running, add the parsley and chop. Add the red pepper flakes, water, 2 teaspoons olive oil, and the vinegar through the feed tube. Process to form a sauce, stopping to scrape sides of bowl down once or twice. It will not be smooth. (Or, if making by hand, chop parsley and garlic together, and mix in the red pepper flakes, water, olive oil, and vinegar.)

2. Place the chicken between 2 pieces of plastic wrap or foil and pound with a meat mallet or bottom of a heavy skillet to 1/4-inch thickness.

3. Heat remaining 2 teaspoons oil in a nonstick skillet over high heat. Add the chicken and brown 2 minutes, turn, and brown 2 more minutes. A meat thermometer inserted into chicken should read 165°F.

4. Remove skillet from the heat and spoon the sauce over the chicken. Cover with a lid and let sit 2 minutes. Add salt and pepper to taste.

*Exchanges/Food Choices: 5 lean protein, 2 fat*
*Per serving: Calories 300, Calories from Fat 130, Total Fat 14 g, Saturated Fat 2.5 g, Monounsaturated Fat 8 g, Cholesterol 125 mg, Sodium 105 mg, Potassium 830 mg, Total Carbohydrate 4 g, Dietary Fiber 2 g, Sugars 0 g, Protein 40 g, Phosphorus 390 mg*

# Red Pepper and Tomato Penne

Serves: 2 / Serving Size: 3/4 cup pasta, 1 cup vegetables

> 1/4 pound whole-wheat penne or other short-cut pasta (about 1 1/4 cups)
> 2 teaspoons olive oil
> 2 medium tomatoes, cut into 1-inch cubes (about 2 cups)
> 1 medium red bell pepper, cut into 1-inch pieces (about 1 1/2 cups)
> 2 medium garlic cloves, crushed
> Salt and freshly ground black pepper, to taste

1. Fill a large saucepan with 3 quarts water and bring to a boil. Add the pasta and boil 9 minutes. Meanwhile, add olive oil to the same skillet used to cook the chicken, and place over medium-high heat.

2. Add the tomatoes, red pepper, and garlic to skillet. Sauté 5 minutes. Remove vegetables to a large bowl.

3. When penne is cooked, drain in a colander and add to the bowl. Toss well, and add salt and pepper to taste.

*Exchanges/Food Choices: 3 starch, 1 vegetable, 1 fat*
*Per serving: Calories 310, Calories from Fat 50, Total Fat 6 g, Saturated Fat 1 g,*
*Monounsaturated Fat 3.5 g, Cholesterol 0 mg, Sodium 15 mg, Potassium 710 mg,*
*Total Carbohydrate 55 g, Dietary Fiber 6 g, Sugars 9 g, Protein 10 g, Phosphorus 175 mg*

## Shopping List:

1 bunch parsley
1 bottle red pepper flakes
1 bottle cider vinegar
3/4 pound boneless, skinless chicken breasts
1 package whole-wheat penne or other short-cut pasta
2 medium tomatoes
1 medium red bell pepper

## Staples:

Garlic
Olive oil
Salt and black peppercorns

## Helpful Hint:

■ Garlic is used in both recipes. Prepare both portions together and divide according to recipes.

## Shop Smart:

■ If buying sauce, look for chimichurri sauce with 90 calories, 9.5 g fat, and 33 mg sodium per tablespoon (Example: Badia Chimichurri Steak Sauce).

# Island Chicken and Papaya with Pigeon Peas and Rice

*Flavors of the sunny Caribbean Islands fill this chicken dish. Pigeon peas are used in some island recipes. They are a legume similar in size to green peas. You can find canned pigeon peas in some markets, or you can substitute frozen green peas.*

## Countdown:

- Prepare all ingredients.
- Start rice.
- Make chicken.
- Finish rice.

## Island Chicken and Papaya

Serves: 2 / Serving Size: 5 ounces chicken, 2 tablespoons sauce with fruit

| | |
|---|---|
| 3/4 pound boneless, skinless chicken breasts | 1 teaspoon ground ginger |
| 1 small papaya | Pinch cayenne pepper |
| 1 tablespoon orange marmalade | Sugar substitute equivalent to 1 teaspoon sugar |
| 1/4 cup fresh lime juice | 2 teaspoons canola oil |
| 1/2 teaspoon ground nutmeg | 1/2 cup chopped fresh cilantro |

1. Remove visible fat from chicken and cut into 1-inch cubes.
2. Peel papaya and cut in half. Remove seeds and cut into 1-inch cubes. Measure out 1/2 cup cubes and set aside. Keep rest for another use.
3. Place marmalade, lime juice, nutmeg, ginger, cayenne pepper, and sugar substitute in a small bowl and mix well. Set aside.
4. Heat oil in a nonstick skillet over medium-high heat and brown the chicken cubes on all sides, about 2 minutes.
5. Add papaya cubes and toss 1–2 minutes. Add marmalade sauce and sauté until chicken is cooked through, about 3–4 minutes, stirring several times during the cooking. A meat thermometer inserted into chicken should read 165°F.
6. Divide between 2 dinner plates and sprinkle with cilantro.

*Exchanges/Food Choices: 1 fruit, 5 1/2 lean protein*
*Per serving: Calories 300, Calories from Fat 80, Total Fat 9 g, Saturated Fat 1.5 g, Monounsaturated Fat 4 g, Cholesterol 125 mg, Sodium 95 mg, Potassium 780 mg, Total Carbohydrate 15 g, Dietary Fiber 2 g, Sugars 10 g, Protein 39 g, Phosphorus 380 mg*

# Pigeon Peas and Rice

Serves: 2 / Serving Size: 1 cup rice/vegetable mixture

> 2 teaspoons canola oil
> 1/2 cup long-grain white rice
> 2 cups fat-free, low-sodium chicken stock
> 1/2 cup canned pigeon peas (rinsed and drained) or frozen green peas
> Salt and freshly ground black pepper, to taste

1. Heat oil in a saucepan over medium-high heat.

2. Add rice. Sauté 1 minute. Add chicken stock and bring to a boil.

3. Reduce heat to low, cover, and simmer 15 minutes. Liquid should be absorbed.

4. Add peas and cook 1 minute to warm peas through. Add salt and pepper to taste.

*Exchanges/Food Choices: 2 1/2 starch, 1 fat*
*Per serving: Calories 260, Calories from Fat 45, Total Fat 5 g, Saturated Fat 0 g,*
*Monounsaturated Fat 3 g, Cholesterol 0 mg, Sodium 150 mg, Potassium 420 mg,*
*Total Carbohydrate 43 g, Dietary Fiber 2 g, Sugars 2 g, Protein 10 g, Phosphorus 210 mg*

## Shopping List:

3/4 pound boneless, skinless chicken breasts
1 small papaya
1 jar orange marmalade
2 limes
1 bottle ground nutmeg
1 bottle ground ginger
1 bottle cayenne pepper
1 bunch cilantro
1 can pigeon peas

## Staples:

Sugar substitute
Canola oil
Long-grain white rice
Fat-free, low-sodium chicken stock
Salt and black peppercorns

## Helpful Hints:

■ Pineapple cubes can be substituted for papaya.
■ Make sure your bottles of dried herbs and spices are less than 6 months old.

## Shop Smart:

■ Look for fat-free, low-sodium chicken stock or broth with 20 calories per cup and about 150 mg sodium per cup.

# Jamaican Jerk Chicken and Quinoa with Coconut and Spinach

*Bring the taste of Jamaica to your kitchen. Jerking is an ancient Jamaican method for preserving and cooking meat. The meat is marinated and slowly cooked over allspice wood. This recipe uses a dry-rub marinade to create the flavors of jerk cooking without spending hours cooking on a barbecue. Use the jerk seasoning recipe provided here or buy one at the market.*

## Countdown:

- Make jerk seasoning and rub it on chicken.
- While chicken marinates, make side dish.
- Sauté chicken.

## Jamaican Jerk Chicken

Serves: 2 / Serving Size: 5 ounces chicken

> 1 tablespoon frozen diced onion, defrosted
> 1 teaspoon dried thyme
> 2 teaspoons sugar
> 1 teaspoon freshly ground black pepper
> 1/4 teaspoon salt
> 1/8 teaspoon ground nutmeg
> 1/8 teaspoon ground allspice
> 3/4 pound boneless, skinless chicken breasts
> 2 teaspoons canola oil

1. Mix onion with the thyme, sugar, black pepper, salt, nutmeg, and allspice.
2. Remove visible fat from the chicken and spoon the jerk seasoning over both sides of chicken. Let marinate while making side dish.
3. Heat oil in a nonstick skillet over low heat and add the chicken. Cover with a lid and gently sauté 5 minutes, turn, and sauté 5 more minutes. A meat thermometer inserted into chicken should read 165°F. Slice and serve with quinoa dish.

*Exchanges/Food Choices: 5 1/2 lean protein, 1/2 fat*
*Per serving: Calories 270, Calories from Fat 80, Total Fat 9 g, Saturated Fat 1.5 g,*
*Monounsaturated Fat 4 g, Cholesterol 125 mg, Sodium 370 mg, Potassium 600 mg,*
*Total Carbohydrate 6 g, Dietary Fiber <1 g, Sugars 5 g, Protein 39 g, Phosphorus 365 mg*

# Quinoa with Coconut and Spinach

Serves: 2 / Serving Size: 1 cup

1/2 cup quinoa
1 1/4 cups water
2 tablespoons unsweetened shredded coconut
2 cups washed, ready-to-eat spinach
Salt and freshly ground black pepper, to taste

1. Place quinoa in a colander or sieve with small openings and run cold water over the grains.

2. Place the quinoa and water in a saucepan. Bring to a boil over high heat. Reduce heat to medium, cover with a lid, and cook 10 minutes. All of the water should be absorbed. If the pan runs dry before the quinoa is cooked, add more water, or if the water is not absorbed, boil until it is absorbed.

3. Add the coconut and spinach. Cook 1–2 minutes or until the spinach wilts. Add salt and pepper to taste.

*Exchanges/Food Choices: 2 starch, 1/2 fat*
*Per serving: Calories 190, Calories from Fat 35, Total Fat 4 g, Saturated Fat 1.5 g, Monounsaturated Fat 1 g, Cholesterol 0 mg, Sodium 40 mg, Potassium 410 mg, Total Carbohydrate 31 g, Dietary Fiber 4 g, Sugars 2 g, Protein 7 g, Phosphorus 210 mg*

## Shopping List:

1 package frozen diced onion
1 bottle dried thyme
1 bottle ground nutmeg
1 bottle ground allspice
3/4 pound boneless, skinless chicken breasts
1 package quinoa
1 package unsweetened shredded
   coconut
1 bag washed, ready-to-eat spinach

## Staples:

Sugar
Salt and black peppercorns
Canola oil

## Helpful Hints:

- Frozen, unsweetened, shredded coconut can be used if packaged dried coconut is unavailable. It does not need to be defrosted before use.
- A quick way to defrost the onion is to place it in a sieve and run hot tap water over it. Squeeze out extra liquid.
- Sauté the chicken on low heat to keep the spices from burning.
- Make sure your bottles of dried herbs and spices are less than 6 months old.

# Mexican Orange Chicken with Green Pepper Rice

*Chicken sautéed in a savory orange sauce is an unusual, tangy Mexican dish. Rice tossed with green peppers makes a simple side dish.*

## Countdown:

- Make rice.
- While rice cooks, prepare chicken ingredients.
- Complete rice.
- Cook chicken.

### Mexican Orange Chicken

Serves: 2 / Serving Size: 5 ounces chicken, 1/4 cup sauce

| | |
|---|---|
| 1 large orange, divided | 3/4 pound boneless, skinless |
| 3 tablespoons flour | chicken thighs |
| Salt and freshly ground black | 1 teaspoon olive oil |
| pepper, to taste | 1/2 cup chopped red onion |
| | 1 teaspoon minced garlic |

1. Cut 2 thin slices from the orange and reserve for garnish (optional). Squeeze juice from remaining orange to make 1/2 cup juice. Set juice aside.

2. Place flour on a plate and season with salt and pepper to taste.

3. Remove visible fat from chicken and dip into seasoned flour, making sure both sides are coated. Shake off excess flour.

4. Heat olive oil in a medium-size nonstick skillet over medium-high heat. Add the chicken, onion, and garlic. Brown chicken 2 minutes, turn, and brown second side 2 minutes.

5. Remove chicken to a plate, and add salt and pepper to taste. Stir orange juice into skillet, scraping up the brown bits on the bottom of the skillet.

6. Reduce heat to medium and return chicken to skillet. Cover with a lid and cook, gently, for 5 minutes. A meat thermometer inserted into chicken should read 170°F. Serve with rice.

*Exchanges/Food Choices: 1 other carbohydrate, 5 lean protein*
*Per serving: Calories 290, Calories from Fat 90, Total Fat 10 g, Saturated Fat 2 g,*
*Monounsaturated Fat 4 g, Cholesterol 160 mg, Sodium 170 mg, Potassium 620 mg,*
*Total Carbohydrate 16 g, Dietary Fiber 1 g, Sugars 7 g, Protein 35 g, Phosphorus 345 mg*

## Green Pepper Rice

Serves: 2 / Serving Size: 1 cup rice/vegetable mixture

**1/2 cup long-grain white rice**
**2 teaspoons olive oil**
**1 cup diced green bell pepper**
**Salt and freshly ground black pepper, to taste**

1. Bring a large saucepan with 2–3 quarts water to a boil. Add rice and boil, uncovered, about 10 minutes.

2. Test a grain; rice should be cooked through, but not soft. Drain into a colander in the sink.

3. Return rice to the pan and mix in oil and green pepper. Add salt and pepper to taste.

*Exchanges/Food Choices: 2 starch, 1 vegetable, 1 fat*
*Per serving: Calories 220, Calories from Fat 45, Total Fat 5 g, Saturated Fat 0.5 g,*
*Monounsaturated Fat 3.5 g, Cholesterol 0 mg, Sodium 0 mg, Potassium 135 mg,*
*Total Carbohydrate 39 g, Dietary Fiber 1 g, Sugars 1 g, Protein 4 g, Phosphorus 60 mg*

## Shopping List:

1 large orange
3/4 pound boneless, skinless chicken thighs
1 red onion
1 green bell pepper

## Staples:

Flour
Salt and black peppercorns
Olive oil
Minced garlic
Long-grain white rice

## Helpful Hints:

- Any type of onion can be used.
- Use a skillet that's just large enough to fit the chicken in one layer. If the skillet is too large, the sauce will boil away.

# Puerto Rican Chicken and Rice

*This is a simple chicken and rice dish. Puerto Rican sofrito is the secret to its flavor. Sofrito is a seasoning sauce used in many Spanish, Caribbean, and Latin American dishes. The basic ingredients for traditional sofrito are: green bell peppers, culantro (saw-leaf coriander, a relative of cilantro), and ajies dulce (sweet cooking peppers). It's an herbal sauce that adds fragrance and flavor to many Puerto Rican dishes. This is a quick version that uses fresh cilantro and cubanel peppers.*

## Countdown:

- Make sofrito.
- Brown chicken.
- Complete dish.

## Puerto Rican Chicken and Rice

Serves: 2 / Serving Size: 5 ounces chicken, 1 1/2 cups vegetables, 3/4 cup rice

    1/2 cup cubed green bell pepper
    4 medium garlic cloves, peeled
    1 cup peeled and quartered onion
    1/2 cup tomato quarters
    1/2 cup cilantro leaves, plus 2 tablespoons (for garnish)
    1/2 cup seeded, cubed cubanel pepper
    Salt and freshly ground black pepper, to taste
    1 tablespoon olive oil
    2 chicken breasts, bone in and wings removed (about 3/4 pound each)
    1/2 cup long-grain white rice
    1/2 cup water
    1/2 cup beer
    3/4 cup frozen peas
    1 cup sliced sweet pimentos

1. Remove skin from chicken.

2. To make the sofrito, place green bell pepper, garlic, onion, tomato, 1/2 cup cilantro, and cubanel pepper in a blender or food processor. Blend until mixed. Add salt and pepper to taste. Set aside.

3. Heat oil in a large nonstick skillet over medium-high heat. Add chicken and brown on all sides about 5 minutes. Add the rice and sauté 1 minute.

4. Add the water, beer, and sofrito. Bring to a simmer, reduce the heat to medium, cover, and cook 15 minutes. Do not let the liquid come to a boil.

5. Add the peas and pimento. Cook 5 more minutes. A meat thermometer inserted into chicken should read 165°F.

6. Add salt and pepper to taste. Sprinkle remaining 2 tablespoons cilantro on top and serve.

*Exchanges/Food Choices: 4 starch, 5 lean protein, 1/2 fat*
*Per serving: Calories 560, Calories from Fat 110, Total Fat 12 g, Saturated Fat 2 g,*
*Monounsaturated Fat 6 g, Cholesterol 125 mg, Sodium 115 mg, Potassium 1310 mg,*
*Total Carbohydrate 60 g, Dietary Fiber 7 g, Sugars 11 g, Protein 47 g, Phosphorus 520 mg*

## Shopping List: | ## Staples:

Shopping List:
1 green bell pepper
1 tomato
1 bunch cilantro
1 cubanel pepper (or mildly hot pepper)
2 chicken breasts, bone in and wings removed (about 3/4 pound each)
1 bottle beer
1 package frozen peas
1 jar sliced sweet pimentos

Staples:
Garlic
Onion
Salt and black peppercorns
Olive oil
Long-grain white rice

## Helpful Hints:

■ White wine or chicken stock can be substituted for the beer.
■ Cubanel peppers are elongated and light green in color. Any other mildly hot peppers can be used instead.
■ Any type of onion can be used.

# Mediterranean

# Chicken Parmesan with Basil Linguine

*Chicken breasts cooked in a spicy tomato sauce and topped with parmesan cheese is an Italian comfort food that has become one of America's favorite meals.*

## Countdown:

- Place water for pasta on to boil.
- Make chicken dish.
- Cook pasta.

### Chicken Parmesan

Serves: 2 / Serving Size: 5 ounces chicken, 1/2 cup sauce, 1 tablespoon cheese

> 2 tablespoons flour
> Salt and freshly ground black pepper, to taste
> 3/4 pound boneless, skinless chicken breasts
> 2 teaspoons olive oil
> 1 cup low-sugar, low-sodium marinara sauce
> 2 teaspoons minced garlic
> Several drops hot pepper sauce
> 2 tablespoons freshly grated parmesan cheese

1. Add flour to a plate and sprinkle with salt and pepper to taste. Roll the chicken breasts in the flour mixture, making sure all sides are covered. Shake off excess and set aside.

2. Heat oil in a medium-size nonstick skillet over medium-high heat. Add chicken and brown 3 minutes. Turn and brown 3 more minutes.

3. Add marinara sauce, garlic, and hot pepper sauce. Mix to combine ingredients. Bring to a simmer, cover with a lid, and simmer 2 minutes; do not boil. A meat thermometer inserted into chicken should read 165°F.

4. Add salt and pepper to taste. Sprinkle parmesan cheese on top.

> *Exchanges/Food Choices: 1 other carbohydrate, 5 1/2 lean protein, 1 fat*
> *Per serving: Calories 350, Calories from Fat 110, Total Fat 12 g, Saturated Fat 2.5 g, Monounsaturated Fat 5 g, Cholesterol 135 mg, Sodium 200 mg, Potassium 1020 mg, Total Carbohydrate 16 g, Dietary Fiber 3 g, Sugars 7 g, Protein 43 g, Phosphorus 455 mg*

## Basil Linguine

Serves: 2 / Serving Size: 3/4 cup

1/4 pound whole-wheat linguine
2 teaspoons olive oil
1/2 cup snipped basil leaves
Salt and freshly ground black pepper, to taste

1. Bring a large pot filled with 3–4 quarts water to a boil.

2. Add the pasta and cook 3–4 minutes if fresh, 10 minutes if dried, or according to package instructions. Remove 2 tablespoons cooking water to a bowl and set aside.

3. Drain pasta. Add the olive oil to the reserved water and mix. Add pasta and basil to bowl and toss well. Add salt and pepper to taste.

4. Divide between 2 dinner plates, and spoon the chicken and sauce on top.

*Exchanges/Food Choices: 2 starch, 1 fat*
*Per serving: Calories 240, Calories from Fat 45, Total Fat 5 g, Saturated Fat 1 g,*
*Monounsaturated Fat 3.5 g, Cholesterol 0 mg, Sodium 5 mg, Potassium 140 mg,*
*Total Carbohydrate 43 g, Dietary Fiber 5 g, Sugars 2 g, Protein 9 g, Phosphorus 150 mg*

## Shopping List:

3/4 pound boneless, skinless chicken breasts
1 bottle low-sugar, low-sodium marinara sauce
1 piece parmesan cheese
1 package whole-wheat linguine
1 bunch basil

## Staples:

Flour
Salt and black peppercorns
Olive oil
Minced garlic
Hot pepper sauce

## Helpful Hints:

- Any type of low-sugar, low-sodium tomato-based sauce can be used.
- Any variety of whole-wheat pasta can be used.
- Snip washed basil leaves with a scissors.

# Chicken Piccata with Spaghettini

*Piccata is a lemon and white wine sauce used to flavor thinly sliced meat. For this dinner, thin chicken cutlets are cooked in the sauce with added mushrooms and capers.*

## Countdown:

- Put water on for pasta to boil.
- Make chicken.
- Cook pasta.

## Chicken Piccata

Serves: 2 / Serving Size: 5 ounces chicken, 1/2 cup vegetables, 1 tablespoon sauce

> 3 tablespoons flour, divided
> 3 tablespoons water
> Salt and freshly ground black pepper, to taste
> 3/4 pound boneless, skinless chicken breast cutlets (1/2 inch thick)
> 2 teaspoons olive oil
> 1 cup sliced mushrooms
> 1 teaspoon minced garlic
> 1/2 cup dry white wine
> 2 tablespoons fresh lemon juice
> 2 tablespoons drained capers
> 1 tablespoon chopped parsley

1. Mix 1 tablespoon flour with the water and set aside.

2. Place remaining 2 tablespoons flour on a plate, and sprinkle with salt and pepper to taste. Add chicken and roll in the flour, making sure all sides are coated with flour. Shake off excess flour.

3. Heat oil in a nonstick skillet over medium-high heat. Add the chicken and brown 2 minutes per side. A meat thermometer inserted into chicken should read 165°F. Transfer to a plate, and add the mushrooms and garlic to the skillet. Sauté 2 minutes or until mushrooms are soft. Spoon mushrooms over chicken.

4. Add the white wine and lemon juice to the skillet, scraping up the brown bits in the bottom of the skillet. Stir the reserved flour and water, and add to the skillet. Bring to a simmer. Cook until the sauce is thickened, about 3–4 minutes. Add the capers and parsley to the sauce, and spoon over the chicken.

5. Serve the chicken over the spaghettini.

*Exchanges/Food Choices: 1/2 other carbohydrate, 1 vegetable, 5 1/2 lean protein, 1 fat*
*Per serving: Calories 340, Calories from Fat 80, Total Fat 9 g, Saturated Fat 1.5 g,*
*Monounsaturated Fat 4.5 g, Cholesterol 125 mg, Sodium 320 mg, Potassium 770 mg,*
*Total Carbohydrate 11 g, Dietary Fiber 1 g, Sugars 2 g, Protein 41 g, Phosphorus 415 mg*

## Spaghettini

Serves: 2 / Serving Size: 3/4 cup

> **1/4 pound whole-wheat spaghettini**
> **3 teaspoons olive oil**
> **Salt and freshly ground black pepper, to taste**

1. Bring a large saucepan filled with water to a boil. Add the spaghettini and boil 8–10 minutes or until the spaghettini is tender but still firm.

2. Remove 2 tablespoons cooking water to a bowl. Add the olive oil to the bowl and mix well. Drain spaghettini. Add the drained spaghettini, and salt and pepper to taste.

*Exchanges/Food Choices: 2 1/2 starch, 1 1/2 fat*
*Per serving: Calories 260, Calories from Fat 70, Total Fat 8 g, Saturated Fat 1 g,*
*Monounsaturated Fat 5 g, Cholesterol 0 mg, Sodium 5 mg, Potassium 125 mg,*
*Total Carbohydrate 43 g, Dietary Fiber 5 g, Sugars 2 g, Protein 8 g, Phosphorus 145 mg*

## Shopping List:

3/4 pound boneless, skinless chicken
   breast cutlets
1 package sliced mushrooms
1 bottle dry white wine
2 lemons
1 bottle capers
1 bunch parsley
1 package whole-wheat spaghettini

## Staples:

Flour
Salt and black peppercorns
Olive oil
Minced garlic

## Helpful Hint:

■ Chicken breasts can be used. Pound them flat to about 1/2 inch thick.

# Chicken Ragout with Mushroom Rice

*Chicken and vegetables in a rich tomato sauce brings memories of Italian slow-cooked stews. This is a quick version that captures those same flavors without costing you hours in the kitchen. It's served with a mushroom and rice side dish.*

## Countdown:

- Prepare ingredients.
- Make rice.
- Make chicken dish.

## Chicken Ragout

Serves: 2 / Serving Size: 5 ounces chicken, 3/4 cup vegetables, 2 tablespoons sauce

> 2 teaspoons olive oil
> 3/4 pound boneless, skinless chicken thighs, cut into 1-inch pieces
> Salt and freshly ground black pepper, to taste
> 1 cup sliced onion
> 2 teaspoons minced garlic
> 1 tomato, cut into 8 wedges
> 1 cup low-sodium, no-sugar-added, diced tomatoes
> 1/2 cup red wine
> 2 tablespoons chopped parsley (optional)

1. Heat oil in a large nonstick skillet over medium-high heat. Add chicken to the skillet and brown the chicken on all sides, about 2 minutes.

2. Remove to a plate, and sprinkle with salt and pepper to taste.

3. Add onion to the skillet and sauté 2 minutes. Add the garlic, tomato wedges, diced tomatoes, and wine. Bring to a simmer and cook 5 minutes. Return chicken to skillet and cook another 3–4 minutes. A meat thermometer inserted into chicken should read 170°F.

4. Remove to 2 plates and sprinkle with parsley (optional).

> *Exchanges/Food Choices: 1/2 other carbohydrate, 2 vegetable, 5 lean protein, 1 fat*
> *Per serving: Calories 360, Calories from Fat 110, Total Fat 12 g, Saturated Fat 2.5 g, Monounsaturated Fat 6 g, Cholesterol 160 mg, Sodium 190 mg, Potassium 1060 mg, Total Carbohydrate 17 g, Dietary Fiber 4 g, Sugars 8 g, Protein 36 g, Phosphorus 400 mg*

# Mushroom Rice

Serves: 2 / Serving Size: 1 cup rice/vegetable mixture

**1/4 pound sliced mushrooms**
**1 package microwave brown rice (to make 1 1/2 cups cooked)**
**1 teaspoon olive oil**
**Salt and freshly ground black pepper, to taste**

1. Place mushrooms in a microwave-safe bowl and microwave on high 1 minute.

2. Remove mushrooms and microwave rice according to package instructions. Measure out 1 1/2 cups rice and set aside any remaining rice for another meal.

3. Add rice to mushrooms along with oil and salt and pepper. Mix and serve.

*Exchanges/Food Choices: 2 starch, 1 vegetable, 1/2 fat*
*Per serving: Calories 200, Calories from Fat 35, Total Fat 4 g, Saturated Fat 0.5 g,*
*Monounsaturated Fat 2 g, Cholesterol 0 mg, Sodium 10 mg, Potassium 250 mg,*
*Total Carbohydrate 36 g, Dietary Fiber 3 g, Sugars 2 g, Protein 6 g, Phosphorus 170 mg*

## Shopping List:

3/4 pound boneless, skinless chicken thighs
1 tomato
1 container low-sodium, no-sugar-added, diced tomatoes
1 bottle red wine
1 bunch parsley (optional)
1/4 pound sliced mushrooms
1 package microwave brown rice

## Staples:

Olive oil
Salt and black peppercorns
Onion
Minced garlic

## Helpful Hints:

■ I find that the low-sodium diced tomatoes in shelf-stable cartons have a real tomato flavor. Any type of onion can be used.
■ A quick way to chop parsley is to snip the leaves with a scissors.

## Shop Smart:

■ Look for low-sodium, no-sugar-added, diced tomatoes with 41 calories, 0.3 g fat, 0.04 g saturated fat, and 24 mg sodium per cup.

# Chicken Tricolore with Spicy Potatoes

*Top sautéed chicken with three different-colored greens for a surprising dinner. It makes a colorful topping for the chicken. Sautéing the greens for a minute enhances the flavor yet still allows the greens to retain a bit of crunch. Preparing the potatoes takes a few extra minutes. Microwaved brown rice can be used instead. Measure out 3/4 cup cooked rice per person.*

## Countdown:

- Marinate chicken.
- Microwave potatoes.
- Make chicken.
- Use same skillet used for chicken to cook greens and to sauté potatoes.

## Chicken Tricolore

Serves: 2 / Serving Size: 5 ounces chicken, 1 1/2 cups salad, 2 tablespoons dressing

> 3/4 pound boneless, skinless chicken breast cutlets (1/2 inch thick)
> 1/4 cup balsamic vinegar
> Vegetable oil cooking spray
> 2 teaspoons olive oil
> 2 teaspoons minced garlic
> 4 cups washed, ready-to-eat greens
>     (including radicchio, romaine, and/or bibb lettuce)
> Salt and freshly ground black pepper, to taste

1. Remove visible fat from chicken.
2. Pour vinegar into resealable bag or bowl and add chicken. Let stand 10 minutes, turning once during that time.
3. Remove chicken from marinade and wipe dry with a paper towel. Discard the marinade.
4. Heat a medium-size nonstick skillet over medium-high heat and spray with cooking spray. Add chicken. Cook chicken 3 minutes, turn, and cook 3 more minutes. Add salt and pepper to taste. Remove chicken to a plate. A meat thermometer inserted into chicken should read 165°F.

---

*Exchanges/Food Choices: 1 vegetable, 5 lean protein, 1 fat*
*Per serving: Calories 290, Calories from Fat 100, Total Fat 11 g, Saturated Fat 2 g,*
*Monounsaturated Fat 6 g, Cholesterol 125 mg, Sodium 90 mg, Potassium 830 mg,*
*Total Carbohydrate 6 g, Dietary Fiber 2 g, Sugars 2 g, Protein 40 g, Phosphorus 400 mg*

5. Heat olive oil in the same skillet. Add garlic and sauté 1 minute. Add salad and toss in pan about 30 seconds. Salad should be warm but remain firm. Add salt and pepper, and spoon salad over chicken.

## Spicy Potatoes

Serves: 2 / Serving Size: 1 cup

**1 pound red potatoes**
**1 tablespoon olive oil**
**1/4 teaspoon cayenne pepper**
**Vegetable oil cooking spray**
**Salt and freshly ground black pepper, to taste**

1. Wash but do not peel potatoes, and slice into thin french fries (1/4-inch-thick strips).

2. Mix oil and cayenne in a medium-size bowl and toss potatoes in oil, making sure to coat all of the potatoes.

3. Cover bowl with a plate or plastic wrap and microwave on high 5 minutes. Remove from microwave.

4. Raise heat to high in the skillet used for greens and spray with vegetable oil cooking spray. Add potatoes and toss about 2–3 minutes or until crisp. Add salt and pepper to taste.

*Exchanges/Food Choices: 2 starch, 1 fat*
*Per serving: Calories 240, Calories from Fat 80, Total Fat 9 g, Saturated Fat 1 g,*
*Monounsaturated Fat 6 g, Cholesterol 0 mg, Sodium 45 mg, Potassium 1040 mg,*
*Total Carbohydrate 37 g, Dietary Fiber 4 g, Sugars 3 g, Protein 4 g, Phosphorus 140 mg*

## Shopping List:

3/4 pound boneless, skinless chicken breast cutlets
1 package washed, ready-to-eat greens including radicchio, romaine, and/or bibb lettuce
1 pound red potatoes
1 bottle cayenne pepper

## Staples:

Balsamic vinegar
Vegetable oil cooking spray
Olive oil
Minced garlic
Salt and black peppercorns

## Helpful Hints:

■ Look for washed, ready-to-eat greens with radicchio, romaine, and other colorful leaves.

■ Any type of potato can be used.

■ Use a resealable plastic bag for marinating. To turn meat over, simply flip over the bag. Using a bag will also save you from having to wash a bowl.

# Gorgonzola Chicken Scaloppini with Fresh Linguine and Sweet Pimentos

*Tangy gorgonzola sauce dresses chicken cutlets in this dish. Gorgonzola is a blue-veined, cow's milk cheese that takes its name from a town in Lombardy. A domestic gorgonzola works very well in this recipe.*

## Countdown:

- Place water for linguine on to boil.
- Prepare all ingredients.
- Make linguine.
- Make chicken.

## Gorgonzola Chicken Scaloppini

Serves: 2 / Serving Size: 5 ounces chicken, 1/4 cup sauce

3 tablespoons flour
Salt and fresh ground black pepper, to taste
3/4 pound boneless, skinless chicken breast cutlets (1/2 inch thick)
Olive oil cooking spray
1/2 cup skim milk
3 tablespoons crumbled gorgonzola cheese
2 tablespoons chopped fresh parsley

1. Place flour on a plate, and season with salt and pepper to taste. Dip the chicken into the flour, making sure both sides are coated. Shake off any extra flour.

2. Heat a small nonstick skillet over medium-high heat and spray with olive oil cooking spray. Add the chicken. Brown 3 minutes, turn over, and brown second side 3 minutes.

3. A meat thermometer inserted into chicken should read 165°F. Transfer to a serving dish and sprinkle with salt and pepper to taste.

4. Add the milk to the skillet and scrape up the brown bits in the bottom of the pan. Cook for about 30 seconds. Immediately add the gorgonzola cheese and stir to melt the cheese; make the mixture into a smooth sauce. Taste for seasoning and add pepper if needed. The cheese should provide enough salt.

5. Remove skillet from heat. Return the chicken to the skillet and turn over in the sauce to warm through. Serve chicken with sauce spooned on top. Scatter parsley over chicken.

*Exchanges/Food Choices: 1/2 other carbohydrate, 5 1/2 lean meat, 1/2 fat*
*Per serving: Calories 300, Calories from Fat 80, Total Fat 9 g, Saturated Fat 3 g,*
*Monounsaturated Fat 3 g, Cholesterol 135 mg, Sodium 300 mg, Potassium 700 mg,*
*Total Carbohydrate 8 g, Dietary Fiber 0 g, Sugars 3 g, Protein 43 g, Phosphorus 470 mg*

## Fresh Linguine with Sweet Pimentos

Serves: 2 / Serving Size: 1 cup pasta/vegetable mixture

**4 ounces fresh spinach linguine**
**2 tablespoons water (reserved from cooking pasta)**
**1/2 teaspoon olive oil**
**3/4 cup drained sweet pimento, cut into 1/4-inch strips**
**Salt and freshly ground black pepper, to taste**

1. Place a large saucepan with 3–4 quarts water on to boil.
2. Add linguine and boil 3 minutes if fresh, 9 minutes if dried. Drain pasta, reserving 2 tablespoons cooking water. Add reserved water to drained pasta. Add oil, sliced pimento, and salt and pepper. Toss well.

*Exchanges/Food Choices: 3 starch*
*Per serving: Calories 240, Calories from Fat 20, Total Fat 2 g, Saturated Fat 0 g,*
*Monounsaturated Fat 1 g, Cholesterol 0 mg, Sodium 15 mg, Potassium 240 mg,*
*Total Carbohydrate 46 g, Dietary Fiber 3 g, Sugars 4 g, Protein 8 g, Phosphorus 120 mg*

## Shopping List:

3/4 pound boneless, skinless chicken breast cutlets
1 small package crumbled gorgonzola cheese
1 bunch parsley
1 package fresh spinach linguine
1 jar sweet pimento

## Staples:

Flour
Salt and black peppercorns
Olive oil cooking spray
Skim milk
Olive oil

## Helpful Hints:

■ Any type of blue-veined cheese can be used. Look for crumbled blue-veined cheese in the dairy section of the supermarket.
■ Any type of linguine can be used.
■ Use a nonstick skillet that's just large enough to fit the chicken in one layer. If the skillet is too big, the sauce will evaporate while cooking.

# Grilled Chicken with Greek Tomato Salad and Brown Rice

*Fresh tomatoes, green bell pepper, and cucumbers create a bright salad that is topped with a grilled chicken breast in this dinner. The salad's crunchy texture contrasts with the juicy chicken.*

## Countdown:

- Prepare ingredients.
- Marinate chicken.
- Make rice.
- Grill chicken.
- Complete dish.

## Grilled Chicken with Greek Tomato Salad

Serves: 2 / Serving Size: 5 ounces chicken, 1 3/4 cups salad, 1 tablespoon dressing

> 1 tablespoon olive oil
> 2 tablespoons fresh lemon juice
> 1/2 teaspoon dried oregano
> Salt and freshly ground black pepper, to taste
> 1 1/4 cups coarsely chopped ripe tomatoes
> 1 cup coarsely chopped green bell pepper
> 1 cup coarsely chopped peeled cucumber
> 8 black pitted olives
> 3/4 pound boneless, skinless chicken breasts

1. Combine olive oil, lemon juice, oregano, and salt and pepper in a medium-size bowl.
2. Place the chicken in a 1-quart plastic bag and pour half of oil mixture over the chicken. Seal the bag. Marinate the chicken 15 minutes.
3. In a second bowl, combine the tomatoes, bell pepper, cucumber, and black olives. Pour the remaining half of the olive oil mixture over the vegetables and set aside.
4. Preheat grill and remove chicken from plastic bag. Grill chicken 5 minutes per side, brushing with the marinade several times. A meat thermometer inserted into chicken should read 165°F.

5. Remove chicken to a cutting board and let rest 5 minutes. Divide the tomato salad between 2 dinner plates. Cut chicken into slices and arrange on top of the salad.

*Exchanges/Food Choices: 2 vegetable, 5 lean protein, 1 1/2 fat*
*Per serving: Calories 320, Calories from Fat 130, Total Fat 14 g, Saturated Fat 2 g,*
*Monounsaturated Fat 8 g, Cholesterol 125 mg, Sodium 210 mg, Potassium 1050 mg,*
*Total Carbohydrate 10 g, Dietary Fiber 3 g, Sugars 5 g, Protein 40 g, Phosphorus 410 mg*

## Brown Rice

Serves: 2 / Serving Size: 3/4 cup

**1 package microwave brown rice**
   **(to yield at least 1 1/2 cups cooked rice)**
**1 teaspoon olive oil**
**Salt and freshly ground black pepper, to taste**

1. Cook rice according to package instructions. Measure 1 1/2 cups and set aside any remaining rice for another dinner.
2. Add the olive oil, and salt and pepper to taste. Mix and serve with the chicken.

*Exchanges/Food Choices: 2 starch, 1/2 fat*
*Per serving: Calories 180, Calories from Fat 30, Total Fat 3.5 g, Saturated Fat 0.5 g,*
*Monounsaturated Fat 2 g, Cholesterol 0 mg, Sodium 10 mg, Potassium 65 mg,*
*Total Carbohydrate 34 g, Dietary Fiber 3 g, Sugars <1 g, Protein 4 g, Phosphorus 120 mg*

## Shopping List:

2 lemons
1 bottle dried oregano
1/2 pound ripe tomatoes
1 green bell pepper
1 cucumber
1 container black pitted olives
3/4 pound boneless, skinless chicken breasts
1 package microwave brown rice

## Staples:

Olive oil
Salt and black peppercorns

## Helpful Hints:

■ The chicken can be made on an outdoor grill, stove-top grill, or sautéed in a skillet.
■ The vegetables can be coarsely chopped using a food processor. Pulse only a few times to prevent them from becoming too processed.
■ Make sure your bottles of dried herbs and spices are less than 6 months old.

# Mediterranean Chicken with Sautéed Fresh Corn

*Tender chicken coated with French Herbes de Provence and served over a bed of baby spinach salad makes a quick dish with the flavors of Provence.*

*Herbes de Provence is a mixture of dried herbs that are grown in the South of France. The assortment usually contains marjoram, rosemary, sage, summer savory, thyme, and lavender. It can be found in some supermarkets. If Herbes de Provence is difficult to find, use equal amounts of dried sage and thyme for the recipe instead.*

## Countdown:
- Sauté chicken.
- Sauté corn.

## Mediterranean Chicken

Serves: 2 / Serving Size: 5 ounces chicken, 1 cup sauce mixture

> 3/4 pound boneless, skinless chicken breasts
> 4 tablespoons Herbes de Provence
> 3 teaspoons olive oil, divided
> 2 tablespoons red wine vinegar
> 2 teaspoons Dijon mustard
> 2 tablespoons water
> Salt and freshly ground black pepper, to taste
> 4 cups washed, ready-to-eat baby spinach leaves

1. Remove visible fat from chicken and rub with Herbes de Provence, making sure to coat both sides.

2. Heat 2 teaspoons olive oil in a nonstick skillet over medium-high heat. Sauté chicken 2 minutes, turn, and sauté 2 more minutes.

3. Remove from heat, cover with a lid, and let sit 10 minutes. A meat thermometer inserted into chicken should read 165°F.

4. Meanwhile, whisk vinegar and mustard together in a salad bowl. Add remaining 1 teaspoon olive oil and water; whisk until smooth. Add salt and pepper to taste. Add spinach and toss well.

5. Divide spinach between 2 dinner plates. Slice chicken into strips and arrange them in the center of the salad. Spoon pan juices over chicken.

*Exchanges/Food Choices: 1 vegetable, 5 1/2 lean protein, 1 fat*
*Per serving: Calories 300, Calories from Fat 110, Total Fat 12 g, Saturated Fat 2 g,*
*Monounsaturated Fat 6 g, Cholesterol 125 mg, Sodium 260 mg, Potassium 970 mg,*
*Total Carbohydrate 6 g, Dietary Fiber 4 g, Sugars <1 g, Protein 41 g, Phosphorus 410 mg*

# Sautéed Fresh Corn

Serves: 2 / Serving Size: 1 cup

> 4 ears fresh corn on the cob OR 3 cups corn kernels
> 1 teaspoon olive oil
> Salt and freshly ground black pepper, to taste

1. Remove husk and silk from corn. Slice the kernels off the cob.

2. Heat the olive oil in a nonstick skillet over medium-high heat and add the corn. Cover and sauté for 4–5 minutes. Remove lid and cook for 1–2 minutes, shaking the pan until the mixture is practically dry and some of the kernels are starting to brown. Remove from heat and spoon onto plate with chicken. Add salt and pepper to taste.

*Exchanges/Food Choices: 2 1/2 starch, 1/2 fat*
*Per serving: Calories 200, Calories from Fat 35, Total Fat 4 g, Saturated Fat 0.5 g,*
*Monounsaturated Fat 2 g, Cholesterol 0 mg, Sodium 5 mg, Potassium 440 mg,*
*Total Carbohydrate 42 g, Dietary Fiber 4 g, Sugars 5 g, Protein 6 g, Phosphorus 145 mg*

## Shopping List:

3/4 pound boneless, skinless chicken breasts
1 bottle Herbes de Provence
1 bottle red wine vinegar
1 jar Dijon mustard
1 bag washed, ready-to-eat baby spinach leaves
4 ears fresh corn on the cob

## Staples:

Olive oil
Salt and black peppercorns

## Helpful Hints:

- Regular spinach can be used if baby leaves are unavailable.
- Balsamic vinegar can be used instead of red wine vinegar.
- To save time, use a reduced-fat vinaigrette instead of making a dressing.
- Frozen corn can be substituted for fresh.
- Make sure your bottles of dried herbs and spices are less than 6 months old.

# Moroccan Spiced Chicken with Spinach and Lentils

*This dish captures the flavors of North Africa with fragrant spices, and it tastes even better the next day. If you have time, make double the recipe and save half for another quick meal. Lentils take 20 minutes to cook and do not need to be soaked.*

## Countdown:

- Start lentils.
- While lentils cook, prepare remaining ingredients.
- Make chicken.

### Moroccan Spiced Chicken

Serves: 2 / Serving Size: 5 ounces chicken, 1/2 cup vegetable mixture

> 1 tablespoon olive oil
> 3/4 pound boneless, skinless chicken thighs, cut into 1-inch cubes
> 2 cups frozen diced onion, defrosted
> 2 medium garlic cloves, crushed
> 1 medium tomato, cut into 8 wedges
> 1 teaspoon ground cinnamon
> 2 teaspoons ground cumin
> 1/8 teaspoon salt
> 1/8 teaspoon freshly ground black pepper
> 2 tablespoons water
> 2 tablespoons chopped cilantro

1. Heat oil in a medium-size nonstick skillet over high heat. Add the chicken cubes and brown for 2 minutes, turning the cubes to make sure all sides are browned.

2. Remove chicken to a plate. Add the onion, garlic, tomato, cinnamon, cumin, salt, and black pepper. Cook 1 minute to release the juices in the dried spices.

3. Add water and return chicken to skillet. Cover with a lid and cook 2–3 minutes. A meat thermometer inserted into chicken should read 170°F. Sprinkle with salt and pepper to taste. Serve over the lentils, and sprinkle cilantro on top.

*Exchanges/Food Choices: 3 vegetable, 5 lean protein, 1 fat*
*Per serving: Calories 340, Calories from Fat 140, Total Fat 15 g, Saturated Fat 3 g,*
*Monounsaturated Fat 8 g, Cholesterol 160 mg, Sodium 340 mg, Potassium 910 mg,*
*Total Carbohydrate 18 g, Dietary Fiber 5 g, Sugars 8 g, Protein 36 g, Phosphorus 385 mg*

## Spinach and Lentils

Serves: 2 / Serving Size: 1 1/4 cups lentil/vegetable mixture

**2 1/2 cups water**
**1/2 cup dried lentils**
**4 cups washed, ready-to-eat spinach**
**Salt and freshly ground black pepper, to taste**

1. Bring water to a boil in a large saucepan. Add the lentils and bring the water back to a boil. Cover and boil 15 minutes. Add 1/4 cup more water if lentils become dry while cooking.

2. Add the spinach and cook another 5 minutes or until lentils are soft. Add salt and pepper to taste.

3. Divide between 2 dinner plates and spoon chicken and sauce on top.

*Exchanges/Food Choices: 2 starch, 1 vegetable*
*Per serving: Calories 180, Calories from Fat 10, Total Fat 1 g, Saturated Fat 0 g,*
*Monounsaturated Fat 0 g, Cholesterol 0 mg, Sodium 50 mg, Potassium 790 mg,*
*Total Carbohydrate 31 g, Dietary Fiber 16 g, Sugars 1 g, Protein 14 g, Phosphorus 245 mg*

## Shopping List:

3/4 pound boneless, skinless chicken thighs
1 package frozen diced onion
1 medium tomato
1 bottle ground cinnamon
1 bottle ground cumin
1 bunch cilantro
1 package dried lentils
1 bag washed, ready-to-eat spinach

## Staples:

Olive oil
Garlic
Salt and black peppercorns

## Helpful Hints:

- A quick way to chop cilantro is to snip the leaves from the stems with a scissors.
- A quick way to defrost the onion is to place it in a sieve and run hot tap water over it. Squeeze out extra liquid.
- Make sure your bottles of dried herbs and spices are less than 6 months old.

# Penne Puttanesca with Italian Salad

*Penne pasta in a zesty tomato sauce flavored with olives and capers is a traditional Italian dish. Arugula, red radicchio, and basil leaves make a colorful Italian salad.*

## Countdown:

- Place water for pasta on to boil.
- Make Penne Puttanesca.
- Make salad.

### Penne Puttanesca

Serves: 2 / Serving Size: 5 ounces chicken, 3/4 cup pasta, 1/2 cup sauce, 1 tablespoon cheese

> 1/4 pound whole-wheat penne pasta
> Olive oil cooking spray
> 2 teaspoons minced garlic
> 3/4 pound boneless, skinless chicken breasts, cut into 1/2-inch cubes
> 1 cup canned, low-sodium tomato sauce
> 1/2 cup water
> 2 tablespoons drained capers
> 8 pitted black olives
> Salt and freshly ground black pepper, to taste
> 2 tablespoons freshly grated parmesan cheese

1. Bring a large pot filled with 3–4 quarts water to a boil. Add penne and cook 10 minutes or according to package instructions.

2. Meanwhile, heat a nonstick skillet over medium-high heat and spray with olive oil cooking spray. Add garlic and chicken, and sauté 4–5 minutes.

3. Add tomato sauce, water, capers, and olives. Blend well. Simmer 2 minutes. A meat thermometer inserted into chicken should read 165°F.

4. Drain pasta and add to skillet. Toss to coat pasta with sauce.

5. Remove from heat. Add salt and pepper to taste, and sprinkle parmesan cheese on top.

*Exchanges/Food Choices: 3 starch, 1 vegetable, 5 1/2 lean protein, 1/2 fat*
*Per serving: Calories 520, Calories from Fat 100, Total Fat 11 g, Saturated Fat 2.5 g,*
*Monounsaturated Fat 4.5 g, Cholesterol 130 mg, Sodium 540 mg, Potassium 1140 mg,*
*Total Carbohydrate 55 g, Dietary Fiber 5 g, Sugars 7 g, Protein 50 g, Phosphorus 545 mg*

# Italian Salad

Serves: 2 / Serving Size: 2 1/2 cups salad, 1 tablespoon dressing

> 2 cups radicchio leaves
> 2 cups fresh arugula, washed
> 1 cup fresh basil, washed
> 2 tablespoons reduced-fat Italian dressing

1. Wash radicchio leaves and tear into bite-size pieces. Place in a bowl with the arugula and basil. Add dressing and toss well.

*Exchanges/Food Choices: 1 vegetable*
*Per serving: Calories 30, Calories from Fat 15, Total Fat 1.5 g, Saturated Fat 0 g, Monounsaturated Fat 0 g, Cholesterol 0 mg, Sodium 20 mg, Potassium 240 mg, Total Carbohydrate 4 g, Dietary Fiber <1 g, Sugars 1 g, Protein 2 g, Phosphorus 35 mg*

## Shopping List:

1 package whole-wheat penne pasta
3/4 pound boneless, skinless chicken breasts
1 can low-sodium tomato sauce
1 bottle capers
1 container black olives
1 small piece parmesan cheese
1 head radicchio
1 package arugula
1 bunch basil

## Staples:

Olive oil cooking spray
Minced garlic
Salt and black peppercorns
Reduced-fat Italian dressing

## Helpful Hints:

- Any type of short-cut pasta such as fusilli (corkscrew) can be used.
- Any type of olive can be used.

## Shop Smart:

- Look for low-sodium tomato sauce with 70 calories, 0.5 g fat, and 27 mg sodium per cup.

# Rosemary-Garlic Chicken with Crunchy Cucumber Rice

*Chicken tenders gently sautéed and served with fresh mint rice is a quick, delicious dinner. This chicken dish works best with a light tomato sauce made from fresh tomatoes. Ripe plum tomatoes are the best type to use for this dinner.*

## Countdown:
- Make rice and set aside.
- Make chicken.

### Rosemary-Garlic Chicken
Serves: 2 / Serving Size: 5 ounces chicken, 3/4 cup vegetables

> 3/4 pound chicken breast tenders
> 3 teaspoons olive oil
> Salt and freshly ground black pepper, to taste
> 2 cups diced ripe plum tomatoes
> 2 medium garlic cloves, crushed
> 1/2 tablespoon dried rosemary

1. Remove visible fat from chicken and cut into 1-inch cubes.

2. Heat oil in a medium nonstick skillet over medium-high heat. Add chicken pieces. Brown on all sides for 2 minutes. Add salt and pepper to taste.

3. Reduce heat to medium, and add tomatoes, garlic, and rosemary. Sauté 5 minutes. A meat thermometer inserted into chicken should read 165°F. Add salt and pepper to taste.

*Exchanges/Food Choices: 2 vegetable, 5 lean protein, 1 fat*
*Per serving: Calories 310, Calories from Fat 110, Total Fat 12 g, Saturated Fat 2 g, Monounsaturated Fat 6 g, Cholesterol 125 mg, Sodium 90 mg, Potassium 1030 mg, Total Carbohydrate 10 g, Dietary Fiber 3 g, Sugars 5 g, Protein 40 g, Phosphorus 410 mg*

# Crunchy Cucumber Rice

Serves: 2 / Serving Size: 1 1/4 cups rice/vegetable mixture

> 1 package microwave brown rice (to yield at least 1 1/2 cups cooked)
> 1 cup peeled and diced cucumber
> 1/2 cup nonfat plain yogurt
> Salt and freshly ground black pepper, to taste
> 1/4 cup chopped fresh mint

1. Microwave rice according to package instructions. Measure out 1 1/2 cups rice and reserve any remaining rice for another meal.

2. Meanwhile, mix cucumber and yogurt together in a serving bowl. Add salt and pepper to taste. Add cooked rice and toss well. Sprinkle mint on top.

*Exchanges/Food Choices: 2 1/2 starch*
*Per serving: Calories 200, Calories from Fat 20, Total Fat 2 g, Saturated Fat 0.5 g,*
*Monounsaturated Fat 0 g, Cholesterol <5 mg, Sodium 50 mg, Potassium 320 mg,*
*Total Carbohydrate 40 g, Dietary Fiber 3 g, Sugars 5 g, Protein 8 g, Phosphorus 190 mg*

## Shopping List:

3/4 pound chicken breast tenders
3 ripe plum tomatoes
1 bottle dried rosemary
1 package microwave brown rice
1 cucumber
1 carton nonfat plain yogurt
1 bunch mint

## Staples:

Olive oil
Salt and black peppercorns
Garlic

## Helpful Hints:

- Boneless, skinless chicken breast can be used instead of chicken tenders.
- To save washing an extra bowl, mix the yogurt sauce for the rice in a serving bowl. Then simply toss the drained rice right in the same bowl.
- A quick way to chop mint is to wash and dry it, and snip the leaves with a scissors right off the stem.

# Spiced Chicken with Tangerine Sauce and Apricot Couscous

*This is a sweet, tangy, and spicy dish. Tangerines add a sweet citrus flavor to this cumin-crusted chicken. Dried apricots add another sweet layer to the couscous side dish.*

## Countdown:

- Prepare ingredients.
- Make couscous and set aside.
- Make chicken.

### Spiced Chicken with Tangerine Sauce

Serves: 2 / Serving Size: 5 ounces chicken, 3/4 cup sauce

2 tablespoons ground cumin
3/4 pound boneless, skinless
    chicken breasts
2 teaspoons olive oil
1/2 cup fat-free, low-sodium
    chicken stock
1/4 cup fresh tangerine juice

1 tablespoon chopped jalapeño
    pepper, seeds and rind
    removed
1 tablespoon Dijon mustard
1 tangerine broken into segments
2 tablespoons chopped cilantro
    (optional)

1. Sprinkle cumin over both sides of chicken.
2. Heat oil in a medium-size skillet over medium-high heat. Add chicken and brown 2 minutes. Turn and brown 2 more minutes.
3. Remove chicken to a plate. Increase heat under skillet to high and add chicken stock; reduce 1 minute. Whisk in the tangerine juice, jalapeño pepper, and mustard to make a smooth sauce.
4. Reduce heat to medium and return chicken to skillet. Cover and gently simmer 5 minutes, turning chicken once during that time. A meat thermometer inserted into chicken should read 165°F.
5. Remove chicken and divide between 2 dinner plates. Add the tangerine segments to the skillet and toss in the sauce. Add salt and pepper to taste. Spoon sauce and tangerine segments over the chicken, and sprinkle cilantro on top (optional).

*Exchanges/Food Choices: 1 fruit, 5 1/2 lean protein, 1/2 fat*
*Per serving: Calories 320, Calories from Fat 100, Total Fat 11 g, Saturated Fat 1.5 g,*
*Monounsaturated Fat 5 g, Cholesterol 125 mg, Sodium 320 mg, Potassium 940 mg,*
*Total Carbohydrate 13 g, Dietary Fiber 2 g, Sugars 8 g, Protein 42 g, Phosphorus 450 mg*

## Apricot Couscous

Serves: 2 / Serving Size: 1 cup couscous mixture

> 3/4 cup water
> 2 teaspoons olive oil
> 1/2 cup whole-wheat couscous
> 2 cups washed, ready-to-eat spinach
> 2 tablespoons dried apricots, cut into 1-inch pieces
> Salt and freshly ground black pepper, to taste

1. Bring water and olive oil to a boil. Remove from the heat, add couscous, and stir. Add spinach and apricots and cover with a lid. Let stand 5 minutes. Add salt and pepper to taste.

*Exchanges/Food Choices: 2 1/2 starch, 1 fat*
*Per serving: Calories 230, Calories from Fat 45, Total Fat 5 g, Saturated Fat 0.5 g,*
*Monounsaturated Fat 3.5 g, Cholesterol 0 mg, Sodium 30 mg, Potassium 330 mg,*
*Total Carbohydrate 40 g, Dietary Fiber 3 g, Sugars 5 g, Protein 7 g, Phosphorus 95 mg*

## Shopping List:

1 bottle ground cumin
3/4 pound boneless, skinless chicken breasts
3 tangerines
1 jalapeño pepper
1 jar Dijon mustard
1 bunch cilantro (optional)
1 package whole-wheat couscous
1 package washed, ready-to-eat spinach
1 package dried apricots

## Staples:

Olive oil
Fat-free, low-sodium chicken stock
Salt and freshly ground black pepper

## Helpful Hints:

- Regular couscous can be used instead of whole-wheat couscous.
- A quick way to chop cilantro is to snip the leaves with a scissors.
- Squeeze juice from tangerines for the small amount needed in the recipe.
- Make sure your bottles of dried herbs and spices are less than 6 months old.

## Shop Smart:

- Look for fat-free, low-sodium chicken stock or broth with 20 calories per cup and about 150 mg sodium per cup.

# Italian Meat Loaf with Hot Pepper Lentils

*This meat loaf recipe is juicy, light, and served with a tomato-mushroom sauce. The meat loaves bake on a baking sheet. They bake faster this way.*

## Countdown:

- Preheat oven to 400°F.
- Start lentils.
- Make meat loaf.

### Italian Meat Loaf

Serves: 2 / Serving Size: 5 ounces chicken, 1/4 cup sauce

> 3/4 pound ground, white-meat-only chicken
> 1 teaspoon fennel seeds
> 2 tablespoons plain bread crumbs
> 1/2 cup frozen diced onion, defrosted
> 1 teaspoon minced garlic
> 1 tablespoon balsamic vinegar
> Salt and freshly ground black pepper, to taste
> 1 egg white
> Olive oil cooking spray
> 1/2 cup sliced mushrooms
> 1/2 cup low-sodium pasta sauce

1. Preheat oven to 400°F. Line a baking sheet with foil and place in the oven while it warms.

2. Mix ground chicken, fennel seeds, bread crumbs, onion, garlic, and balsamic vinegar together. Add salt and pepper to taste. Add the egg white and blend together.

3. Remove baking tray from oven, spray with cooking spray. Shape chicken into 2 loaves (about 5 x 3 inches) on the sheet. Spread mushrooms and pasta sauce on top. Bake 15 minutes. A meat thermometer inserted into chicken should read 165°F.

> *Exchanges/Food Choices: 1/2 other carbohydrate, 2 vegetable, 5 lean protein*
> *Per serving: Calories 320, Calories from Fat 70, Total Fat 8 g, Saturated Fat 1.5 g, Monounsaturated Fat 2.5 g, Cholesterol 125 mg, Sodium 190 mg, Potassium 960 mg, Total Carbohydrate 17 g, Dietary Fiber 3 g, Sugars 7 g, Protein 43 g, Phosphorus 430 mg*

## Hot Pepper Lentils

Serves: 2 / Serving Size: 3/4 cup

> 1 cup fat-free, low-sodium chicken stock
> 1 1/2 cups water
> 1/2 cup frozen diced onion, defrosted
> 1/8 teaspoon crushed red pepper flakes
> 1/2 cup lentils
> 1 tablespoon olive oil
> 2 teaspoons dried oregano
> Salt and freshly ground black pepper, to taste

1. Bring chicken stock and water to a boil in a medium-size saucepan over high heat. Add onion and crushed red pepper. Slowly pour lentils into boiling liquid so that it continues to boil.

2. Reduce heat to a simmer and cook, covered, for 20 minutes.

3. Check after 10 minutes. If dry, add 1/2 cup water. If liquid is left after 20 minutes, remove lid and boil several minutes until liquid evaporates.

4. Add olive oil, oregano, and salt and pepper, and serve with the meat loaf.

*Exchanges/Food Choices: 2 starch, 1/2 other carbohydrate 1 1/2 fat*
*Per serving: Calories 250, Calories from Fat 60, Total Fat 7 g, Saturated Fat 1 g,*
*Monounsaturated Fat 5 g, Cholesterol 0 mg, Sodium 85 mg, Potassium 770 mg,*
*Total Carbohydrate 33 g, Dietary Fiber 16 g, Sugars 3 g, Protein 15 g, Phosphorus 290 mg*

## Shopping List:

3/4 pound ground, white-meat-only chicken
1 bottle fennel seeds
1 container plain bread crumbs
1 package frozen diced onion
1 container sliced mushrooms
1 bottle low-sodium pasta sauce
1 bottle crushed red pepper flakes
1 package dried lentils
1 bottle dried oregano

## Staples:

Minced garlic
Balsamic vinegar
Salt and black peppercorns
Eggs
Olive oil cooking spray
Fat-free, low-sodium chicken stock
Olive oil

## Helpful Hints:

- A quick way to defrost the onion is to place it in a sieve and run hot tap water over it. Squeeze out extra liquid. Frozen onions are used in both recipes. Prepare both servings at the same time and divide according to recipes.
- Make sure your bottles of dried herbs and spices are less than 6 months old.

(continued on page 88)

**Italian Meat Loaf with Hot Pepper Lentils** (continued from page 87)

## Shop Smart:

- Look for fat-free, low-sodium chicken stock or broth with 20 calories per cup and about 150 mg sodium per cup.

- Look for low-sodium pasta sauce with 130 calories, less than 4.0 g fat, and 80 mg sodium per cup.

- Look for ground chicken made from chicken breast meat only. If the label just says "ground chicken," then skin, fat, and dark meat may have been added.

# Asian/Indian

# Chicken Satay with Thai Peanut Sauce and Broccoli Rice

*I have fond memories of the enticing aroma of skewered meat cooking on small grills in the street markets of South East Asia. These skewers of small cubes or strips of seafood or meat are called satays, and they're usually served with a spicy peanut sauce.*

## Countdown:

- Preheat broiler and baking tray.
- Start rice.
- While rice cooks, prepare remaining ingredients.
- Make peanut sauce.
- Broil chicken satay.

## Chicken Satay with Thai Peanut Sauce

Serves: 2 / Serving Size: 5 ounces chicken, 1 3/4 tablespoons sauce

    3/4 pound boneless, skinless chicken breasts,
        cut into 1/2-inch-thick x 4-inch-long strips
    4 8-inch metal skewers
    Olive oil cooking spray
    Salt and freshly ground black pepper, to taste
    1 1/2 tablespoons crunchy, no-sugar-added peanut butter
    1 tablespoon low-sodium soy sauce
    1 tablespoon rice wine vinegar
    6 drops hot pepper sauce
    1 teaspoon cornstarch
    2 tablespoons water

1. Move an oven rack so that it is about 4 inches from the broiler heat. Preheat broiler. Line a baking tray with foil and place under broiler to heat.

2. Thread the chicken strips onto the skewers. (Threading in a wave pattern allows for more even cooking.) Remove baking sheet from oven and place skewers on sheet. Spray chicken with olive oil cooking spray. Sprinkle with salt and pepper to taste. Place under broiler for 3 minutes.

3. Remove chicken from broiler. A meat thermometer inserted into chicken should read 165°F. Place skewers on 2 dinner plates.

4. To make Thai Peanut Sauce, mix peanut butter, soy sauce, and vinegar

together in a microwave-safe bowl until blended with a smooth consistency. Add hot pepper sauce. Mix cornstarch and water together in a separate container, then blend into the peanut butter mixture. Microwave on high 1 minute, or, alternatively, place the mixture in a saucepan over medium heat and cook until sauce is thick (about 2 minutes). If sauce becomes too thick, add another tablespoon water to make it a thick-but-pourable consistency. Spoon the sauce over the chicken.

*Exchanges/Food Choices: 6 lean protein, 1 fat*
*Per serving: Calories 310, Calories from Fat 120, Total Fat 13 g, Saturated Fat 2 g,*
*Monounsaturated Fat 5 g, Cholesterol 125 mg, Sodium 350 mg, Potassium 690 mg,*
*Total Carbohydrate 5 g, Dietary Fiber 1 g, Sugars 1 g, Protein 42 g, Phosphorus 410 mg*

## Broccoli Rice

Serves: 2 / Serving Size: 1 1/4 cups rice/vegetable mixture

**1 cup water**
**1 cup 10-minute brown rice**
**1/4 pound broccoli florets (about 1 2/3 cups)**
**2 teaspoons canola oil**
**Salt and freshly ground black pepper, to taste**

1. Place water in a medium-size saucepan and bring to a boil over high heat. Add the rice and broccoli, cover with a lid, and simmer 5 minutes.

2. Remove from the heat and let sit 5 minutes. Add the canola oil and salt and pepper. Toss well.

*Exchanges/Food Choices: 2 starch, 1 vegetable, 1 fat*
*Per serving: Calories 210, Calories from Fat 50, Total Fat 6 g, Saturated Fat 0 g,*
*Monounsaturated Fat 3 g, Cholesterol 0 mg, Sodium 20 mg, Potassium 230 mg,*
*Total Carbohydrate 36 g, Dietary Fiber 2 g, Sugars 0 g, Protein 6 g, Phosphorus 120 mg*

## Shopping List:      Staples:

3/4 pound boneless, skinless chicken breasts    8-inch metal skewers
1 jar crunchy peanut butter (no sugar added)    Olive oil cooking spray
1 bottle low-sodium soy sauce    Salt and black peppercorns
1 bottle rice wine vinegar    Hot pepper sauce
1 package 10-minute brown rice    Cornstarch
1 package broccoli florets    Canola oil

## Helpful Hints:

■ Rice wine vinegar can be bought in the Asian section of the supermarket, or substitute 1/2 tablespoon water mixed with 1/2 tablespoon distilled white vinegar.

■ Buy peanut butter that does not have added sugar.

# Curry-Kissed Chicken with Rice and Carrots

*A dusting of curry flavors this simple chicken dish. The curry powder sold in supermarkets is a blend of about 15 herbs, spices, and seeds. This type of powder loses its flavor quickly. If you have curry powder that is more than 6 months old, buy a new bottle. It will add more flavors to the dish.*

## Countdown:

- Place water for rice on to boil.
- Assemble ingredients for chicken.
- Cook rice.
- While rice cooks, make chicken.

### Curry-Kissed Chicken

Serves: 2 / Serving Size: 5 ounces chicken, 3 tablespoons sauce

> 1 1/2 tablespoons curry powder
> 3/4 pound chicken breast tenders
> Olive oil cooking spray
> Salt and freshly ground black pepper, to taste
> 1/3 cup water
> 3 tablespoons apricot jam
> 1 1/2 tablespoons light cream
> 1 scallion, sliced

1. Place curry powder on a plate. Turn the chicken tenders in the curry powder, making sure all sides are coated.

2. Heat a nonstick skillet over medium-high heat and spray with olive oil cooking spray. Add the chicken tenders and sauté 3 minutes per side. Add salt and pepper to taste. A meat thermometer inserted into chicken should read 165°F.

3. Remove chicken to a clean plate. Add the water and apricot jam to the skillet and simmer 30 seconds, stirring to melt jam. Add cream and simmer 2 minutes to thicken sauce. Add salt and pepper to taste.

4. Spoon sauce over chicken. Sprinkle scallions on top.

*Exchanges/Food Choices: 1 1/2 other carbohydrate, 5 lean protein*
*Per serving: Calories 340, Calories from Fat 90, Total Fat 10 g, Saturated Fat 2.5 g,*
*Monounsaturated Fat 3.5 g, Cholesterol 135 mg, Sodium 100 mg, Potassium 680 mg,*
*Total Carbohydrate 23 g, Dietary Fiber 3 g, Sugars 14 g, Protein 40 g, Phosphorus 390 mg*

## Rice and Carrots

Serves: 2 / Serving Size: 1 cup rice/vegetable mixture

> 1 cup water
> 1 cup 10-minute brown rice (to yield at least 1 1/2 cups cooked rice)
> 1/2 cup shredded carrots
> 2 teaspoons olive oil
> Salt and freshly ground black pepper, to taste

1. Bring water to a boil in a large saucepan over high heat. Stir in rice and return to a boil. Reduce heat to medium, cover, and simmer 5 minutes.

2. Remove from heat and stir in shredded carrots. Cover and let stand 5 minutes. Add oil, and salt and pepper to taste. Fluff with a fork.

*Exchanges/Food Choices: 2 starch, 1 fat*
*Per serving: Calories 200, Calories from Fat 50, Total Fat 6 g, Saturated Fat 0.5 g,*
*Monounsaturated Fat 3.5 g, Cholesterol 0 mg, Sodium 25 mg, Potassium 130 mg,*
*Total Carbohydrate 36 g, Dietary Fiber 3 g, Sugars 1 g, Protein 4 g, Phosphorus 90 mg*

## Shopping List:

1 bottle curry powder
3/4 pound chicken breast tenders
1 jar apricot jam
1 small carton light cream
1 bunch scallions
1 package 10-minute brown rice
1 bag shredded carrots

## Staples:

Olive oil cooking spray
Salt and black peppercorns
Olive oil

## Helpful Hints:

■ If chicken tenders are not available, use boneless, skinless chicken breasts and cut them into 3-inch strips.
■ Make sure your bottles of dried herbs and spices are less than 6 months old.

# "Dead Easy" Chicken with Chinese Rice

*"Dead easy" is how TV cooking personality and chef Ken Hom described this chicken recipe to me. Chinese five-spice powder is one of the ingredients that flavors this meal. It's a pungent mixture used in Chinese cooking that includes cinnamon, cloves, fennel seed, star anise, and Szechwan peppercorns.*

## Countdown:

- Place chicken on to cook.
- Make rice.

### "Dead Easy" Chicken

Serves: 2 / Serving Size: 5 ounces chicken, 1 tablespoon sauce

> 3/4 pound boneless, skinless chicken thighs
> 2 tablespoons flour
> 1/2 cup fat-free, low-sodium chicken stock
> 3 tablespoons rice wine vinegar
> 1 teaspoon Chinese five-spice powder
> 5 large garlic cloves, peeled
> 1 1/2 tablespoons low-sodium soy sauce
> 1/2 cup water
> 1 teaspoon canola oil

1. Remove visible fat from chicken. Place flour on a plate and roll chicken in flour. Shake off excess flour.

2. Mix chicken stock, vinegar, Chinese five-spice, garlic, soy sauce, and water together. Set sauce aside.

3. Heat oil in a wok or skillet over high heat until smoking. Brown chicken on all sides (about 2 minutes).

4. Add sauce and reduce heat to medium. Simmer gently 25 minutes, turning chicken a few times. Liquid should be just at the bubbling stage. The sauce will boil down to a glaze as the chicken cooks.

5. Remove garlic cloves and serve over rice.

*Exchanges/Food Choices: 1/2 other carbohydrate, 5 lean protein, 1/2 fat*
*Per serving: Calories 270, Calories from Fat 90, Total Fat 10 g, Saturated Fat 2 g, Monounsaturated Fat 4 g, Cholesterol 160 mg, Sodium 590 mg, Potassium 590 mg, Total Carbohydrate 7 g, Dietary Fiber <1 g, Sugars 0 g, Protein 37 g, Phosphorus 385 mg*

# Chinese Rice

Serves: 2 / Serving Size: 1 1/2 cups rice/vegetable mixture

**1/2 cup long-grain white rice**
**3/4 cup water**
**6 scallions, sliced (about 1 cup)**
**1 cup fresh bean sprouts**
**1 teaspoon sesame oil**
**Salt and freshly ground black pepper, to taste**

1. Combine rice with water in a medium-size saucepan, cover, and bring to a boil over high heat. Stir, reduce heat to medium, and continue to boil, covered, about 10 minutes.

2. Remove cover and stir to make sure no rice sticks to the bottom. If rice is still very moist, simmer uncovered until only a few drops of moisture remain.

3. Remove from heat. Add scallions, bean sprouts, oil, and salt and pepper. Cover and let rest 10 minutes. Loosen grains before serving.

*Exchanges/Food Choices: 2 starch, 2 vegetable, 1/2 fat*
*Per serving: Calories 220, Calories from Fat 25, Total Fat 2.5 g, Saturated Fat 0 g,*
*Monounsaturated Fat 1 g, Cholesterol 0 mg, Sodium 10 mg, Potassium 260 mg,*
*Total Carbohydrate 43 g, Dietary Fiber 3 g, Sugars 3 g, Protein 6 g, Phosphorus 100 mg*

## Shopping List:

3/4 pound boneless, skinless chicken thighs
1 bottle rice wine vinegar
1 bottle Chinese five-spice powder
1 bottle low-sodium soy sauce
1 bunch scallions
1 package fresh bean sprouts
1 bottle sesame oil

## Staples:

Flour
Fat-free, low-sodium chicken stock
Garlic
Canola oil
Long-grain white rice
Salt and black peppercorns

## Helpful Hints:

- Chinese five-spice powder can be found in the spice section of the market.
- White vinegar diluted with an equal amount of water can be used instead of rice wine vinegar.
- Microwave rice can be used instead of long-grain white rice in side dish recipe.
- Make sure your bottles of dried herbs and spices are less than 6 months old.

## Shop Smart:

- Look for fat-free, low-sodium chicken stock or broth with 20 calories per cup and about 150 mg sodium per cup.

# Japanese Barbecued Chicken and Mushrooms with Sesame Rice

*These quick, easy, grilled chicken kabobs are made with a sweet Japanese barbecue marinade. The secret to quick and even kabob cooking is to leave a little space on the skewer between pieces of chicken. This way the chicken can cook through on all sides.*

## Countdown:

- Make sauce and marinate chicken and mushrooms.
- Heat stove-top grill.
- Start rice.
- Skewer and cook kabobs.
- Finish rice.

### Japanese Barbecued Chicken and Mushrooms

Serves: 2 / Serving Size: 5 ounces chicken, 1 1/2 cups vegetable/sauce mixture

> Vegetable oil cooking spray
> 1 1/2 tablespoons low-sodium soy sauce
> 2 tablespoons dry sherry
> 2 tablespoons rice wine vinegar
> 2 tablespoons water
> 2 tablespoons sugar
> 3/4 pound boneless, skinless chicken breasts, cut into 1-inch cubes
> 1/4 pound shiitake mushrooms (about 8 mushrooms),
>     thick part of stems removed
> 1 red bell pepper, cut into 2-inch pieces
> 4 large skewers

1. Heat a stove-top grill over high heat. Spray with vegetable oil cooking spray.

2. Mix soy sauce, sherry, vinegar, water, and sugar in a small saucepan. Add chicken, mushrooms, and pepper, and marinate 5 minutes while rice is started.

3. Remove chicken and mushrooms from sauce, making sure to reserve sauce. Place chicken, mushrooms, and red pepper on skewers, alternating ingredients until the skewers are full. Leave at least 1/4-inch space between items.

4. Place skewers on stove-top grill and cook 5 minutes. Turn and cook 5 more minutes. A meat thermometer inserted into chicken should read 165°F.

5. Bring reserved sauce to a boil in saucepan and boil 3 minutes. Serve skewers over Sesame Rice and drizzle sauce on top.

*Exchanges/Food Choices: 1 other carbohydrate, 1 vegetable, 5 lean protein*
*Per serving: Calories 310, Calories from Fat 45, Total Fat 5 g, Saturated Fat 1 g,*
*Monounsaturated Fat 1 g, Cholesterol 125 mg, Sodium 470 mg, Potassium 920 mg,*
*Total Carbohydrate 20 g, Dietary Fiber 2 g, Sugars 16 g, Protein 42 g, Phosphorus 445 mg*

## Sesame Rice

Serves: 2 / Serving Size: 3/4 cup

**1 package microwave brown rice**
  **(to yield at least 1 1/2 cups cooked rice)**
**1 tablespoon sesame oil**
**Salt and freshly ground black pepper, to taste**

1. Cook rice according to package instructions. Measure out 1 1/2 cups rice and set aside any remaining rice for another meal. Add the oil, and salt and pepper to taste.

*Exchanges/Food Choices:  2 starch, 1 1/2 fat*
*Per serving: Calories 220, Calories from Fat 70, Total Fat 8 g, Saturated Fat 1 g,*
*Monounsaturated Fat 3 g, Cholesterol 0 mg, Sodium 10 mg, Potassium 65 mg,*
*Total Carbohydrate 34 g, Dietary Fiber 3 g, Sugars <1 g, Protein 4 g, Phosphorus 120 mg*

## Shopping List:

1 bottle low-sodium soy sauce
1 bottle dry sherry
1 bottle rice wine vinegar
3/4 pound boneless, skinless chicken breasts
1/4 pound shiitake mushrooms
1 red bell pepper
1 package microwave brown rice
1 bottle sesame oil

## Staples:

Vegetable oil cooking spray
Sugar
Skewers
Salt and black peppercorns

## Helpful Hints:

- Any type of mushrooms can be used.
- White vinegar diluted with an equal amount of water can be used instead of rice wine vinegar.
- The skewers can also be cooked in a broiler or on an outdoor grill.
- If using wooden skewers, soak them in water for about 30 minutes before use.

# Kung Pao Chicken with Chinese Noodles

*Spicy, flavorful Kung Pao Chicken is a popular Chinese dish. It's topped with a sauce of garlic, ginger, red chile peppers, and soy sauce. Small red chile peppers have different names and origins. A common type of chile used in this dish is the bird pepper. They are very hot. Dried ones can be found in many supermarkets.*

## Countdown:

- Marinate chicken.
- Make noodles.
- Complete chicken recipe.

### Kung Pao Chicken

Serves: 2 / Serving Size: 2 cups

> 3/4 pound boneless, skinless chicken breasts
> 1 tablespoon low-sodium soy sauce
> 1 tablespoon rice wine vinegar
> 3–4 small dried bird or red chile peppers, chopped (about 1 tablespoon)
> 3 teaspoons minced garlic
> 2 slices fresh ginger, cut into small pieces
> 1 tablespoon hoisin sauce
> 1/2 cup water
> 2 teaspoons sesame oil
> 1/2 pound broccoli florets
> 2 scallions, sliced
> 2 tablespoons dry-roasted, unsalted peanuts

1. Cut chicken into thin slices (about 1/4 inch thick).

2. Mix soy sauce, vinegar, chilies, and garlic together. Place ginger slices in garlic press and squeeze juice into sauce. Add the chicken to the sauce, toss in sauce once or twice, and let stand while preparing remaining ingredients.

3. Remove chicken from marinade. Mix hoisin sauce and water into marinade juices. Set aside.

4. Heat oil in a wok or skillet over high heat, until smoking. Add the chicken and stir-fry 3 minutes.

5. Remove chicken and add the marinade and broccoli to the wok. Stir-fry over high heat 4–5 minutes or until broccoli is cooked.

6. Remove wok from the heat and add the scallions and chicken. Toss well. Spoon over noodles and sprinkle peanuts on top.

*Exchanges/Food Choices: 3 vegetable, 5 1/2 lean protein, 1 1/2 fat*
*Per serving: Calories 380, Calories from Fat 140, Total Fat 15 g, Saturated Fat 2.5 g,*
*Monounsaturated Fat 5 g, Cholesterol 125 mg, Sodium 500 mg, Potassium 1180 mg,*
*Total Carbohydrate 18 g, Dietary Fiber 3 g, Sugars 3 g, Protein 46 g, Phosphorus 510 mg*

## Chinese Noodles

Serves: 2 / Serving Size: 3/4 cup

**1/4 pound Chinese egg noodles**
**2 teaspoons sesame oil**
**Salt and freshly ground black pepper, to taste**

1. Bring a large saucepan filled with water to a boil over high heat. Add the noodles. Boil 1 minute. Drain noodles and place back in saucepan.

2. Add oil, and salt and pepper to taste. Serve with chicken.

*Exchanges/Food Choices: 2 1/2 starch, 1 fat*
*Per serving: Calories 240, Calories from Fat 45, Total Fat 5 g, Saturated Fat 1 g,*
*Monounsaturated Fat 1.5 g, Cholesterol 50 mg, Sodium 10 mg, Potassium 140 mg,*
*Total Carbohydrate 41 g, Dietary Fiber 2 g, Sugars 1 g, Protein 8 g, Phosphorus 135 mg*

## Shopping List:      Staples:

3/4 pound boneless, skinless chicken breasts    Minced garlic
1 bottle low-sodium soy sauce               Salt and black peppercorns
1 bottle rice wine vinegar
1 package small dried bird or red chile
   peppers
1 small piece fresh ginger
1 bottle hoisin sauce
1 bottle sesame oil
1 package broccoli florets
1 bunch scallions
1 bottle dry-roasted, unsalted peanuts
1 package Chinese egg noodles

## Helpful Hints:

- 1/2 teaspoon crushed red pepper can be used instead of bird peppers.
- White vinegar diluted with an equal amount of water can be used instead of rice wine vinegar.

# Mu Shu Chicken Wrap with Chinese Egg Noodles

*This is a quick take on a Chinese classic. It's made with sautéed chicken and shredded cabbage and wrapped in lettuce leaves.*

## Countdown:

- Prepare all ingredients.
- Marinate chicken.
- Place water for noodles on to boil.
- Make noodles.
- Complete chicken dish.

### Mu Shu Chicken Wrap

Serves: 2 / Serving Size: 1 1/2 cups filling mixture

3/4 pound boneless, skinless chicken breast tenders
1 teaspoon minced garlic
1 tablespoon grated fresh ginger
2 tablespoons dry sherry
1 teaspoon sesame oil
2 cups ready-to-eat shredded cabbage
Salt and freshly ground black pepper, to taste
2 tablespoons hoisin sauce
6 large iceberg lettuce leaves

1. Remove visible fat from chicken and cut into strips about 1/4 inch thick.

2. Mix garlic, ginger, and sherry together in a bowl, then add the chicken strips. Set aside.

3. Heat oil in a wok or skillet over high heat and add the cabbage. Stir-fry 2 minutes. Push cabbage to the sides of the pan, and add the chicken and sauce. Stir-fry 3–4 minutes in the center of the pan. Draw in the cabbage and continue to cook 2 minutes. Add salt and pepper to taste.

4. Spread hoisin sauce on lettuce leaves. Add chicken and vegetables. Roll up.

*Exchanges/Food Choices: 2 vegetable, 5 1/2 lean protein, 1/2 fat*
*Per serving: Calories 320, Calories from Fat 70, Total Fat 8 g, Saturated Fat 1.5 g,*
*Monounsaturated Fat 2 g, Cholesterol 125 mg, Sodium 360 mg, Potassium 920 mg,*
*Total Carbohydrate 17 g, Dietary Fiber 4 g, Sugars 8 g, Protein 41 g, Phosphorus 415 mg*

## Chinese Egg Noodles

Serves: 2 / Serving Size: 3/4 cup

> 1/4 pound Chinese egg noodles
> 2 tablespoons dry-roasted, unsalted peanuts
> 2 teaspoons sesame oil

1. Bring a large saucepan filled with water to a boil over high heat. Add the noodles and boil 3 minutes. Drain pasta, reserving 1 tablespoon cooking water in the saucepan.

2. Add the oil to the pan and return the noodles to it. Add the peanuts, and salt and pepper to taste. Toss well.

*Exchanges/Food Choices: 3 starch, 2 fat*
*Per serving: Calories 310, Calories from Fat 110, Total Fat 12 g, Saturated Fat 2 g,*
*Monounsaturated Fat 5 g, Cholesterol 50 mg, Sodium 15 mg, Potassium 200 mg,*
*Total Carbohydrate 43 g, Dietary Fiber 3 g, Sugars 2 g, Protein 10 g, Phosphorus 170 mg*

## Shopping List:

3/4 pound boneless, skinless chicken
   breast tenders
1 small piece fresh ginger
1 bottle dry sherry
1 bottle sesame oil
1 bag ready-to-eat shredded cabbage
1 bottle hoisin sauce
1 head iceberg lettuce
1 package Chinese egg noodles
1 bottle dry-roasted, unsalted peanuts

## Staples:

Minced garlic
Salt and black peppercorns

## Helpful Hints:

- Romaine lettuce leaves can be used instead of iceberg lettuce.
- Angel-hair pasta can be used instead of Chinese egg noodles.
- Ready-to-eat shredded cabbage for coleslaw can be found in the produce section of the market.

# Sesame Chicken with Snow Peas and Rice

*Honey, ginger, and soy sauce lend a sweet and savory flavor to this quick-cooked chicken. A coating of sesame seeds brightens the dish and adds a crunchy texture.*

## Countdown:

- Make chicken.
- While chicken cooks, make rice.

## Sesame Chicken

Serves: 2 / Serving Size: 5 ounces chicken, 1 tablespoon sauce

> 3/4 pound boneless, skinless chicken thighs, opened flat
> 1 tablespoon honey
> 1/4 teaspoon ground ginger
> 2 teaspoons low-sodium soy sauce
> Olive oil cooking spray
> 1 1/2 tablespoons sesame seeds

1. Remove visible fat from chicken.

2. Mix honey, ginger, and soy sauce together; set aside.

3. Heat a nonstick skillet over medium-high heat and spray with olive oil cooking spray. Add the chicken and sauté 5 minutes. Turn chicken and sauté 3 more minutes. A meat thermometer inserted into chicken should read 170°F.

4. Spoon sauce over the chicken and let warm in skillet for about 30 seconds, turning chicken in the sauce to make sure both sides are coated. The sauce will turn thick and provide a sweet and savory coating.

5. Remove to individual dishes and sprinkle sesame seeds on top.

*Exchanges/Food Choices: 1/2 other carbohydrate, 5 lean protein, 1 fat*
*Per serving: Calories 300, Calories from Fat 120, Total Fat 13 g, Saturated Fat 2.5 g,*
*Monounsaturated Fat 5 g, Cholesterol 160 mg, Sodium 340 mg, Potassium 470 mg,*
*Total Carbohydrate 11 g, Dietary Fiber <1 g, Sugars 9 g, Protein 35 g, Phosphorus 365 mg*

# Snow Peas and Rice

Serves: 2 / Serving Size: 1 3/4 cups rice/vegetable mixture

> 3 cups trimmed snow peas (about 12 ounces)
> 1 package microwave brown rice
>   (to yield at least 1 1/2 cups cooked rice)
> 2 teaspoons sesame oil
> Salt and freshly ground black pepper, to taste

1. Place snow peas in a microwave-safe bowl. Microwave on high 2 minutes. Remove from microwave.

2. Add the brown rice to the microwave and cook according to package instructions. Remove and measure out 1 1/2 cups cooked rice. Save any remaining rice for another meal.

3. Add rice to snow peas along with sesame oil. Add salt and pepper to taste. Toss well.

*Exchanges/Food Choices: 2 1/2 starch, 1 fat*
*Per serving: Calories 240, Calories from Fat 50, Total Fat 6 g, Saturated Fat 1 g,*
*Monounsaturated Fat 2.5 g, Cholesterol 0 mg, Sodium 10 mg, Potassium 250 mg,*
*Total Carbohydrate 41 g, Dietary Fiber 5 g, Sugars 4 g, Protein 6 g, Phosphorus 170 mg*

## Shopping List:

3/4 pound boneless, skinless chicken thighs
1 small bottle honey
1 bottle ground ginger
1 bottle low-sodium soy sauce
1 container sesame seeds
1 package snow peas
1 package microwave brown rice
1 bottle sesame oil

## Staples:

Olive oil cooking spray
Salt and black peppercorns

## Helpful Hints:

- Boneless, skinless chicken breasts can be used instead of thighs. A meat thermometer inserted into chicken should read 165°F for the cooked breast meat.
- Look for trimmed snow peas in the produce section of the market.
- Any type of green vegetable such as green beans or broccoli can be used in the rice.

# Stir-Fried Diced Chicken with Cucumbers and Brown Rice

*Garlic, sherry, and hoisin sauce flavor chicken in this quick Chinese stir-fry. The cooking time for the chicken recipe is only 5 minutes. The cucumber gives the dish an intriguing texture and flavor.*

## Countdown:

- Marinate chicken.
- Make rice.
- While chicken marinates, prepare other ingredients.
- Stir-fry chicken.

### Stir-Fried Diced Chicken with Cucumbers

Serves: 2 / Serving Size: 2 cups chicken/vegetable mixture

    1 tablespoon sugar
    1/4 cup dry sherry
    3 teaspoons minced garlic
    1 teaspoon ground ginger
    3/4 pound chicken breast tenders, cut into 1/2-inch cubes
    2 tablespoons cornstarch
    1 tablespoon hoisin sauce
    1 tablespoon water
    1 tablespoon sesame oil
    2 cups peeled cucumber, cut into 1/2-inch cubes
    Salt and freshly ground black pepper, to taste
    2 scallions, sliced

1. Mix sugar, sherry, garlic, and ground ginger together in a bowl or plastic bag. Add chicken and marinate for 10 minutes while you prepare other ingredients.

2. Remove chicken from mixture to a plate, reserving marinade. Sprinkle cornstarch over chicken and toss. Set aside.

3. Mix hoisin sauce and water with the reserved marinade.

4. Heat oil in wok or skillet over high heat. Drain any excess liquid left on the chicken, and add chicken to the wok. Stir-fry 3 minutes. Add cucumber cubes and stir-fry 2 minutes. Remove to a bowl. A meat thermometer inserted into chicken should read 165°F.

5. Add marinade to the wok and cook 2–3 minutes. Pour sauce over chicken and cucumbers, and toss well. Add salt and pepper to taste. Sprinkle with scallions, and spoon over rice.

*Exchanges/Food Choices: 1 1/2 other carbohydrate, 1 vegetable, 5 lean protein, 1 fat*
*Per serving: Calories 410, Calories from Fat 110, Total Fat 12 g, Saturated Fat 2 g,*
*Monounsaturated Fat 4 g, Cholesterol 125 mg, Sodium 220 mg, Potassium 860 mg,*
*Total Carbohydrate 28 g, Dietary Fiber 2 g, Sugars 11 g, Protein 40 g, Phosphorus 415 mg*

## Brown Rice

Serves: 2 / Serving Size: 3/4 cup

**1 package microwave brown rice (to yield at least 1 1/2 cups cooked rice)**
**2 teaspoons sesame oil**
**Salt and freshly ground black pepper, to taste**

1. Microwave rice according to package instructions. Measure out 1 1/2 cups rice and reserve any remaining rice for another meal. Add oil, and salt and pepper to taste. Toss well.

*Exchanges/Food Choices: 2 starch, 1 fat*
*Per serving: Calories 200, Calories from Fat 50, Total Fat 6 g, Saturated Fat 1 g,*
*Monounsaturated Fat 2.5 g, Cholesterol 0 mg, Sodium 10 mg, Potassium 65 mg,*
*Total Carbohydrate 34 g, Dietary Fiber 3 g, Sugars <1 g, Protein 4 g, Phosphorus 120 mg*

## Shopping List:

1 bottle dry sherry
1 bottle ground ginger
3/4 pound chicken breast tenders
1 small bottle hoisin sauce
1 bottle sesame oil
1 cucumber
1 bunch scallions
1 package microwave brown rice

## Staples:

Sugar
Minced garlic
Cornstarch
Salt and black peppercorns

## Helpful Hints:

■ Low-sodium soy sauce can be substituted for the hoisin sauce.
■ Minced garlic can be found in the produce section.
■ For easy stir-frying, place the prepared ingredients on a cutting board or plate in order of use. That way you won't have to look at the recipe once you start to cook.
■ Make sure your wok is very hot before adding the ingredients.
■ A quick way to slice scallions is to snip them with a scissors.

# Wasabi Chicken with Pan-Roasted Ginger, Corn, and Snow Peas

*Spicy wasabi sauce gives pan-seared chicken an Asian flavor. Corn and ginger tossed with snow peas complete this Pacific Rim dinner. Wasabi is the Japanese version of horseradish. It's an Asian root vegetable that is sold in paste and powdered form. The powdered form is mixed with water to form a thick paste. The powder loses its flavor quickly. Make sure you have a fresh bottle. Fresh wasabi root can be found in some Asian stores.*

## Countdown:

- Make chicken.
- While chicken cooks, make sauce.
- Make corn and snow pea dish.

## Wasabi Chicken

Serves: 2 / Serving Size: 5 ounces chicken, 2 tablespoons sauce

> 3 tablespoons reduced-fat mayonnaise
> 3 teaspoons wasabi powder
> 1 teaspoon canola oil
> 3/4 pound boneless, skinless chicken breast cutlets (1/2 inch thick)
> Salt and freshly ground black pepper, to taste

1. Mix mayonnaise with wasabi powder and set aside.

2. Heat oil in a large nonstick skillet over medium-high heat. Add the chicken and sear 3 minutes. Turn and sear the other side for 3 more minutes. Salt and pepper the cooked sides to taste. A meat thermometer inserted into chicken should read 165°F.

3. Remove skillet from heat and place chicken on a plate. Spread the wasabi sauce over the chicken. Cover with another plate or foil to keep warm until the vegetables are ready. Use the same skillet for the side dish.

*Exchanges/Food Choices: 5 1/2 lean protein, 1 1/2 fat*
*Per serving: Calories 310, Calories from Fat 130, Total Fat 14 g, Saturated Fat 2 g,*
*Monounsaturated Fat 4.5 g, Cholesterol 125 mg, Sodium 240 mg, Potassium 590 mg,*
*Total Carbohydrate 3 g, Dietary Fiber <1 g, Sugars <1 g, Protein 39 g, Phosphorus 360 mg*

## Pan-Roasted Ginger, Corn, and Snow Peas

Serves: 2 / Serving Size: 2 cups

> 2 teaspoons canola oil
> 2 cups frozen corn kernels
> 2 cups frozen snow peas
> 1 medium red bell pepper, sliced (about 1 cup)
> 2 teaspoons ground ginger
> Salt and freshly ground black pepper, to taste

1. Add the oil to the nonstick skillet used for the chicken and heat over medium-high heat.

2. Add the corn, snow peas, red pepper, and ground ginger. Toss to coat the vegetables with the oil. Cook 7–8 minutes, turning vegetables over as they cook. Add salt and pepper to taste.

*Exchanges/Food Choices: 1 1/2 starch, 2 vegetable, 1 fat*
*Per serving: Calories 210, Calories from Fat 50, Total Fat 6 g, Saturated Fat 0.5 g,*
*Monounsaturated Fat 3 g, Cholesterol 0 mg, Sodium 10 mg, Potassium 540 mg,*
*Total Carbohydrate 37 g, Dietary Fiber 6 g, Sugars 8 g, Protein 6 g, Phosphorus 140 mg*

## Shopping List:

1 jar reduced-fat mayonnaise
1 bottle wasabi powder
3/4 pound boneless, skinless chicken
　　breast cutlets
1 package frozen corn kernels
1 package frozen snow peas
1 medium red bell pepper
1 bottle ground ginger

## Staples:

Canola oil
Salt and black peppercorns

## Helpful Hints:

- To save washing an extra pan, use the same skillet for the chicken and the vegetables.
- Prepared horseradish can be used instead of wasabi powder.
- Make sure your bottles of dried herbs and spices are less than 6 months old.

# Sandwich Suppers

# Barbecued-Chicken Roll with Peppery Bean Salad

*A juicy, barbecued-chicken sandwich with a bell pepper and bean salad makes an easy sandwich supper. Cumin and chili powder add a kick to the bean and pepper salad.*

## Countdown:

- Make salad.
- Prepare chicken dish.

### Barbecued-Chicken Roll

Serves: 2 / Serving Size: 5 ounces chicken, 2 tablespoons sauce, 1 roll

> 3/4 pound boneless, skinless chicken breast cutlets (1/2 inch thick)
> 1 teaspoon canola oil
> 1/2 cup low-sodium barbecue sauce
> 2 whole-wheat hamburger rolls (1 1/2 ounces each)

1. Cut chicken into thin strips.

2. Heat oil in a nonstick skillet over medium-high heat. Add chicken and sauté 3 minutes, turning the pieces as they cook. Add the barbecue sauce and continue to cook 2–3 minutes to warm the sauce. A meat thermometer inserted into chicken should read 165°F.

3. To serve, slice rolls in half and toast in toaster or regular oven for 2 minutes. Spoon the chicken and sauce on both halves and serve as an open-face sandwich.

*Exchanges/Food Choices: 3 starch, 5 lean protein*
*Per serving: Calories 450, Calories from Fat 80, Total Fat 9 g, Saturated Fat 1.5 g, Monounsaturated Fat 3 g, Cholesterol 125 mg, Sodium 360 mg, Potassium 830 mg, Total Carbohydrate 46 g, Dietary Fiber 3 g, Sugars 25 g, Protein 44 g, Phosphorus 460 mg*

# Peppery Bean Salad

Serves: 2 / Serving Size: 1 1/4 cups salad, 1 tablespoon dressing

- 2 tablespoons reduced-fat oil and vinegar dressing
- 1/2 teaspoon ground cumin
- 1/2 teaspoon chili powder
- 1 medium green bell pepper, sliced (about 2 cups)
- 1/2 cup canned red kidney beans, rinsed and drained
- Salt and freshly ground black pepper, to taste

1. Mix dressing with the ground cumin and chili powder together in a small bowl. Add green pepper and kidney beans. Toss well. Add salt and pepper. Taste for seasoning, adding more cumin, chili powder, or salt and pepper, if needed.

*Exchanges/Food Choices: 1/2 starch, 1 vegetable, 1/2 fat*
*Per serving: Calories 80, Calories from Fat 15, Total Fat 1.5 g, Saturated Fat 0 g, Monounsaturated Fat 0 g, Cholesterol 0 mg, Sodium 90 mg, Potassium 290 mg, Total Carbohydrate 14 g, Dietary Fiber 5 g, Sugars 4 g, Protein 4 g, Phosphorus 70 mg*

## Shopping List:

3/4 pound boneless, skinless chicken breast cutlets
1 bottle low-sodium barbecue sauce
1 package whole-wheat hamburger rolls
1 bottle ground cumin
1 bottle chili powder
1 medium green bell pepper
1 small can red kidney beans

## Staples:

Canola oil
Reduced-fat oil and vinegar dressing
Salt and black peppercorns

## Helpful Hints:

- Look for no-salt-added or low-sodium barbecue sauce.
- Any type of reduced-fat oil and vinegar dressing can be used for the salad.
- To avoid heating up a large oven for 2 rolls, use a toaster oven.
- Make sure your bottles of dried herbs and spices are less than 6 months old.

## Shop Smart:

- Look for low-sodium barbecue sauce with 29 calories, 7 g carbohydrate, and 23 mg sodium per tablespoon.

# Chicken Pita Pocket with Greek Salad

*A chicken pita pocket garnished with a tomato and corn salsa makes a quick and light dinner. Let the supermarket do the work, and doctor up store-bought salsa with frozen corn kernels.*

## Countdown:

- Prepare tomato and corn salsa and set aside to marinate a few minutes.
- Make salad.
- Cook chicken and finish pita pocket.

## Chicken Pita Pocket

Serves: 2 / Serving Size: 3 ounces chicken, 1/4 cup salsa, 1 (2-ounce) pita bread

> 1/4 cup frozen corn kernels, defrosted
> 1/4 cup store-bought tomato salsa
> 2 teaspoons canola oil
> 1/2 pound boneless, skinless chicken breast cutlets (1/2 inch thick)
> Salt and freshly ground black pepper, to taste
> 2 large whole-wheat pita breads (about 6 inches each)

1. Mix corn and salsa together and set aside.

2. Heat oil in a nonstick skillet over medium-high heat. Add chicken and sauté 3 minutes, turn, and sauté 3 more minutes. A meat thermometer inserted into chicken should read 165°F.

3. Remove chicken from skillet, add salt and pepper to taste, and slice into thin strips.

4. Toast pita bread in a toaster oven to warm slightly. Do not let it get too crisp. Cut both pieces of pita bread in half and open pockets. Spoon the chicken into the pockets and top with the salsa.

*Exchanges/Food Choices: 2 1/2 starch, 3 1/2 lean protein, 1/2 fat*
*Per serving: Calories 370, Calories from Fat 80, Total Fat 9 g, Saturated Fat 1.5 g,*
*Monounsaturated Fat 4 g, Cholesterol 85 mg, Sodium 480 mg, Potassium 610 mg,*
*Total Carbohydrate 41 g, Dietary Fiber 6 g, Sugars 2 g, Protein 33 g, Phosphorus 375 mg*

## Greek Salad

Serves: 2 / Serving Size: 2 1/4 cups salad, 1 tablespoon dressing

1 teaspoon dried oregano OR 2 tablespoons fresh oregano leaves
2 tablespoons reduced-fat oil and vinegar dressing
2 cups washed, ready-to-eat lettuce
2 cups peeled and sliced cucumbers
7 green or black olives

1. Mix oregano and vinaigrette dressing in a medium-size salad bowl. Add the lettuce, cucumber, and olives. Toss with dressing.

*Exchanges/Food Choices: 1 vegetable, 1/2 fat*
*Per serving: Calories 50, Calories from Fat 25, Total Fat 3 g, Saturated Fat 0 g,*
*Monounsaturated Fat 1.5 g, Cholesterol 0 mg, Sodium 120 mg, Potassium 350 mg,*
*Total Carbohydrate 6 g, Dietary Fiber 2 g, Sugars 3 g, Protein 2 g, Phosphorus 40 mg*

## Shopping List:

1 package frozen corn kernels
1 jar tomato salsa
1/2 pound boneless, skinless chicken breast cutlets
1 package whole-wheat pita breads
1 bottle dried oregano
1 bag washed, ready-to-eat lettuce
1 cucumber
1 container green or black olives

## Staples:

Canola oil
Salt and freshly ground black pepper
Reduced-fat oil and vinegar dressing

## Helpful Hints:

- A quick way to defrost the corn kernels is to place them in a sieve and run hot tap water over them. Squeeze out extra liquid.
- Fresh corn can be used instead of frozen. Cut the kernels from the corn and microwave on high for 1 minute.
- Make sure your bottles of dried herbs and spices are less than 6 months old.

## Shop Smart:

- Look for whole-wheat pita breads, about 6 inches in diameter, weighing 64 g (a little over 2 ounces), with 170 calories, 1.7 g fat, and 284 mg sodium each.

# Curried Chicken Salad Wrap

*Savor a hint of India with these wraps, which are made with chicken, curry powder, and raisins. The curried chicken salad can also be served over lettuce leaves with a slice of whole-grain bread.*

## Countdown:

- Cook chicken.
- While chicken cooks, prepare remaining ingredients.
- Finish salad and wrap.

### Curried Chicken Salad Wrap

Serves: 2 / Serving Size: 3 ounces chicken, 3/4 cup sauce/vegetable mixture, 1 tortilla

> 1 teaspoon canola oil
> 1/2 pound boneless, skinless chicken breast cutlets (1/2 inch thick)
> Salt and freshly ground black pepper, to taste
> 3 tablespoons reduced-fat mayonnaise
> 1/4 cup nonfat plain yogurt
> 1 teaspoon curry powder
> 1/2 cup sliced celery
> 1/4 cup raisins
> 2 small lettuce leaves
> 2 8-inch whole-wheat tortillas

1. Heat oil in a nonstick skillet over medium-high heat. Add the chicken cutlets and sauté 3 minutes. Turn and sauté 3 more minutes. Add salt and pepper to taste. A meat thermometer inserted into chicken should read 165°F.

2. Remove to a cutting board and cut into 1/4-inch cubes.

3. Mix mayonnaise, yogurt, curry powder, celery, and raisins together in a bowl. Add the cooked chicken, and toss well.

4. Place tortillas on a countertop and place a lettuce leaf in the center of each one. Divide the chicken salad between them. Roll up and place on 2 plates, with the seam side down. Cut in half and serve.

*Exchanges/Food Choices: 3 starch, 4 lean protein, 2 fat*
*Per serving: Calories 500, Calories from Fat 210, Total Fat 23 g, Saturated Fat 3.5 g, Monounsaturated Fat 7 g, Cholesterol 95 mg, Sodium 550 mg, Potassium 780 mg, Total Carbohydrate 44 g, Dietary Fiber 5 g, Sugars 16 g, Protein 32 g, Phosphorus 450 mg*

## Shopping List:

1/2 pound boneless, skinless chicken
    breast cutlets
1 carton nonfat plain yogurt
1 bottle curry powder
1 bunch celery
1 small container raisins
1 small head lettuce
1 package 8-inch whole-wheat tortillas

## Staples:

Canola oil
Salt and black peppercorns
Reduced-fat mayonnaise

## Helpful Hint:

■ Use mild or hot curry powder. The heat is up to you. Make sure the powder is less than 6 months old.

## Shop Smart:

■ Look for whole-wheat tortillas, 8 inches in diameter, weighing 48 g (a little under 2 ounces), with 130 calories, 2 g fat, and 330 mg sodium per tortilla.

# Sloppy Joes
# with Dipping Veggies

*Sloppy Joe's Bar in Key West, Florida, claims that their picadillo recipe
from Havana, Cuba, became the basis for Sloppy Joes sandwiches. Sloppy
Joes are an American staple with as many variations as there are people
who make it. This version is based on the Sloppy Joe's Bar original.*

## Countdown:

- Prepare all ingredients.
- Make vegetables and dip and set aside.
- Make Sloppy Joes.

## Sloppy Joes

Serves: 2 / Serving Size: 5 ounces chicken, 1 cup sauce/vegetable mixture, 1 roll

> 1 teaspoon canola oil
> 3/4 pound ground, white-meat-only chicken
> Salt and freshly ground black pepper, to taste
> 1 cup mushrooms, cut into cubes
> 1 cup frozen diced onion, defrosted
> 1 cup frozen diced green bell pepper, defrosted
> 2 teaspoons minced garlic
> 2 cups low-sodium pasta sauce
> 1 tablespoon distilled white vinegar
> 2 whole-wheat hamburger rolls (about 1 1/2 ounces each)

1. Heat oil in a large nonstick skillet over medium-high heat. Add the ground chicken and sauté 2–3 minutes, breaking up the pieces as they cook.

2. Remove chicken to a plate, and sprinkle with salt and pepper to taste.

3. Add the mushrooms, onion, green pepper, and garlic, and cook 2 minutes. Add the pasta sauce. Cook until the sauce starts to bubble, about 2 minutes. Add the vinegar. Cook 1 minute.

4. Return the ground chicken to the skillet. Cook 2–3 minutes. Add salt and pepper to taste.

5. Toast rolls in a toaster oven or under the broiler. Place them on 2 dinner plates and spoon chicken and sauce on top.

*Exchanges/Food Choices: 2 1/2 starch, 3 vegetable, 5 1/2 lean protein, 1/2 fat
Per serving: Calories 510, Calories from Fat 110, Total Fat 12 g, Saturated Fat 2 g,
Monounsaturated Fat 4 g, Cholesterol 130 mg, Sodium 370 mg, Potassium 1820 mg,
Total Carbohydrate 50 g, Dietary Fiber 10 g, Sugars 21 g, Protein 50 g, Phosphorus 605 mg*

## Dipping Veggies

Serves: 2 / Serving Size: 1 1/4 cups vegetables, 2 tablespoons sauce

2 tablespoons reduced-fat mayonnaise
2 tablespoons low-sodium ketchup
1/2 cup sliced carrots
1 cup celery sticks
1 cup broccoli florets

1. Mix mayonnaise and ketchup together, and divide into 2 small bowls. Set aside.

2. Divide the vegetables between the 2 plates used to serve the Sloppy Joes. Serve the dipping sauce on the side.

*Exchanges/Food Choices: 2 vegetable, 1 fat*
*Per serving: Calories 90, Calories from Fat 45, Total Fat 5 g, Saturated Fat 0.5 g,*
*Monounsaturated Fat 1 g, Cholesterol 0 mg, Sodium 180 mg, Potassium 400 mg,*
*Total Carbohydrate 11 g, Dietary Fiber 2 g, Sugars 7 g, Protein 2 g, Phosphorus 50 mg*

## Shopping List:

3/4 pound ground, white-meat-only chicken
1 package mushrooms
1 package frozen diced onion
1 package frozen diced green bell pepper
1 jar low-sodium pasta sauce
1 small bottle distilled white vinegar
1 package whole-wheat hamburger rolls
   (about 1 1/2 ounces each)
Low-sodium ketchup
1 package sliced carrots
1 package celery sticks
1 package broccoli florets

## Staples:

Canola oil
Salt and black peppercorns
Minced garlic
Reduced-fat mayonnaise

## Helpful Hints:

■ Any type of vegetables can be used for the side dish. Buy ones that are already cut for dipping to save time.

■ A quick way to defrost the onion and green peppers is to place them in a sieve and run hot tap water over them. Squeeze out extra liquid.

## Shop Smart:

■ Look for low-sodium pasta sauce with 130 calories, less than 4 g fat, and 80 mg sodium per cup.

■ Look for low-sodium ketchup with 16 calories and 3 mg sodium per tablespoon.

■ Look for ground chicken made from chicken breast meat only. If the label just says "ground chicken," then skin, fat, and dark meat may have been added.

# Sun-Dried Tomato and Chicken Sandwich

*This sandwich supper is made with tender chicken tenderloins. Sweet sun-dried tomatoes, zippy arugula, and pine nuts add crunch and flavor.*

## Countdown:

- Place sun-dried tomatoes in hot water to reconstitute.
- Prepare remaining ingredients.
- Make sandwich.

### Sun-Dried Tomato and Chicken Sandwich

Serves: 2 / Serving Size: 3 ounces chicken, 1 cup vegetable/sauce mixture, 2 slices bread

> 1/2 cup sun-dried tomatoes (not packed in oil)
> 1 cup hot water
> 1/2 pound boneless, skinless chicken breast tenders
> 2 teaspoons olive oil
> 4 slices multi-grain bread
> 3 tablespoons reduced-fat mayonnaise
> Salt and freshly ground black pepper, to taste
> 2 tablespoons pine nuts
> 1/4 cup fresh basil leaves
> 1 cup baby arugula

1. Cut sun-dried tomatoes in half and place in hot water to reconstitute them. Set aside.

2. Cut chicken tenders in half lengthwise. Heat oil in a nonstick skillet over medium-high heat. Add chicken and sauté 3 minutes. Turn and sauté 3 more minutes. A meat thermometer inserted into chicken should read 165°F.

3. Toast bread slices. Place bread on a countertop and spread mayonnaise over the slices. Divide the chicken in half and place over 2 slices of the bread. Sprinkle with salt and pepper to taste.

4. Drain the tomatoes and squeeze out extra moisture. Place over the chicken. Sprinkle pine nuts on top. Divide the basil and arugula in 2 portions and place over the pine nuts. Close the sandwiches with the remaining 2 toast slices. Cut the sandwiches in half and serve.

*Exchanges/Food Choices: 2 starch, 4 1/2 lean protein, 2 fat*
*Per serving: Calories 460, Calories from Fat 190, Total Fat 21 g, Saturated Fat 3.5 g,*
*Monounsaturated Fat 8 g, Cholesterol 85 mg, Sodium 450 mg, Potassium 1060 mg,*
*Total Carbohydrate 33 g, Dietary Fiber 6 g, Sugars 10 g, Protein 36 g, Phosphorus 415 mg*

## Shopping List:

1 package sun-dried tomatoes (not packed in oil)
1/2 pound boneless, skinless chicken breast tenders
1 loaf multi-grain bread
1 package pine nuts
1 package fresh basil
1 package baby arugula

## Staples:

Olive oil
Reduced-fat mayonnaise
Salt and black peppercorns

## Helpful Hints:

■ Use baby arugula if possible. It has a sweeter flavor.
■ Be sure to use sun-dried tomatoes that are not packed in oil.

# Salad and Soup Suppers

# All-American Chicken Salad Supper

*Cooked white meat chicken breast, plump blueberries, and red bell pepper make this a colorful and patriotic dish. The dressing lightly coats the salad. It is made with yogurt and mayonnaise mixed with prepared horseradish to add a tangy boost to the salad.*

## Countdown:

- Sauté chicken.
- Toast bread.
- Make dressing and finish salad.
- Arrange lettuce, tomatoes, and cucumbers.

## All-American Chicken Salad Supper

Serves: 2 / Serving Size: 5 ounces chicken, 1 1/2 cups vegetable mixture

Olive oil cooking spray
3/4 pound boneless, skinless chicken breast cutlets (1/2 inch thick)
Salt and freshly ground black pepper, to taste
2 slices whole-grain bread
1/4 cup reduced-fat mayonnaise
1/4 cup nonfat plain yogurt
1 tablespoon prepared horseradish
1 cup blueberries
1 cup red bell pepper, cut into 1/2-inch cubes
1/2 cup sliced scallions
2 large wedges iceberg lettuce
1 large tomato, sliced
1/2 cucumber, peeled and sliced
3 tablespoons reduced-fat oil and vinegar dressing

1. Heat a nonstick skillet over medium-high heat and spray with olive oil cooking spray. Add the chicken and sauté 5 minutes. Turn and sauté 3 more minutes. A meat thermometer inserted into chicken should read 165°F. Sprinkle with salt and pepper to taste.

2. Remove chicken to a cutting board and slice into strips about 1/2 inch x 1 inch.

3. Toast bread and spray with olive oil cooking spray. Set aside.

4. In a large bowl, combine mayonnaise, yogurt, and horseradish. Stir chicken, blueberries, red pepper, and scallions into the dressing. Add salt and pepper to taste. Toss well.

5. Place a slice of bread on each plate and spoon salad on top of toast.

6. Place 1 lettuce wedge on each plate. Alternate the tomato and cucumber slices next to the lettuce. Sprinkle with salt and pepper to taste, and drizzle with reduced-fat salad dressing.

*Exchanges/Food Choices: 1 starch, 1 fruit, 2 vegetable, 5 1/2 lean protein, 2 fat*
*Per serving: Calories 530, Calories from Fat 180, Total Fat 20 g, Saturated Fat 3 g,*
*Monounsaturated Fat 6 g, Cholesterol 130 mg, Sodium 470 mg, Potassium 1480 mg,*
*Total Carbohydrate 41 g, Dietary Fiber 9 g, Sugars 21 g, Protein 47 g, Phosphorus 545 mg*

## Shopping List:

3/4 pound boneless, skinless chicken breast cutlets
1 loaf whole-grain bread
1 carton nonfat plain yogurt
1 bottle prepared horseradish
1 container blueberries
1 red bell pepper
1 bunch scallions
1 head iceberg lettuce
1 large tomato
1 cucumber

## Staples:

Olive oil cooking spray
Salt and black peppercorns
Reduced-fat mayonnaise
Reduced-fat oil and vinegar dressing

## Helpful Hints:

■ Any type of berries can be used for the salad.
■ The quickest way to slice scallions is to snip them with a scissors.

# Caribbean Chicken Salad

*This is a very pretty salad with the pineapple, tomatoes, and black beans giving it vivid colors. Allspice coats the chicken. Allspice is a berry with flavors suggesting cinnamon, cloves, and nutmeg, and it appears often in Caribbean cooking.*

## Countdown:

- Start chicken.
- Prepare remaining ingredients.
- Assemble salad.

## Caribbean Chicken Salad

Serves: 2 / Serving Size: 5 ounces chicken, 2 cups salad, 2 tablespoons dressing

> Vegetable oil cooking spray
> 3/4 pound boneless, skinless chicken thighs
> 1 teaspoon ground allspice
> Salt and freshly ground black pepper, to taste
> 4 cups shredded romaine lettuce
> 1/4 cup shredded reduced-fat cheddar cheese
> 1 cup canned black beans, rinsed and drained
> 1 cup fresh pineapple cubes
> 1 cup plum tomatoes, cut into 1/4–1/2-inch pieces
> 1/4 cup reduced-fat oil and vinegar dressing
> 1/2 cup sliced scallions

1. Heat a nonstick skillet over medium-high heat and spray with vegetable oil cooking spray.

2. Remove visible fat from chicken and add chicken to the skillet. Sauté 5 minutes, turn, and sprinkle the cooked side with the allspice and salt and pepper. Sauté 3 more minutes. A meat thermometer inserted into chicken should read 170°F.

3. Remove chicken and cut into 1/2-inch cubes.

4. Place lettuce on a serving platter, sprinkle the cheddar cheese on top, and spoon the black beans, pineapple, and tomatoes over the cheese. Sprinkle the dressing over the salad. Top with the chicken and then the scallions.

> *Exchanges/Food Choices: 1 1/2 starch, 1 fruit, 1 vegetable, 5 1/2 lean protein, 1/2 fat*
> *Per serving: Calories 460, Calories from Fat 120, Total Fat 13 g, Saturated Fat 3 g,*
> *Monounsaturated Fat 5 g, Cholesterol 165 mg, Sodium 410 mg, Potassium 1430 mg,*
> *Total Carbohydrate 42 g, Dietary Fiber 13 g, Sugars 14 g, Protein 47 g, Phosphorus 580 mg*

## Shopping List:

3/4 pound boneless, skinless
  chicken thighs
1 bottle ground allspice
1 package shredded romaine lettuce or
  1 head lettuce
1 package shredded reduced-fat cheddar
  cheese
1 small can black beans
1 container fresh pineapple cubes
2 plum tomatoes
1 bunch scallions

## Staples:

Vegetable oil cooking spray
Salt and black peppercorns
Reduced-fat oil and vinegar dressing

## Helpful Hints:

- Shredded low-fat cheddar cheese can be found in the cheese case. Any type of low-fat cheese can be used.
- A quick way to slice scallions is to snip them with a scissors.
- Make sure your bottles of dried herbs and spices are less than 6 months old.

# Chicken–Sweet Potato Salad

*This is a light chicken and potato salad. The chicken is cooked in the same pan used for the potatoes. It can be made in advance and tastes great the next day.*

## Countdown:

- Place potatoes on to cook.
- Make dressing.
- Sauté chicken when potatoes are removed from pan.
- Complete salad.

## Chicken–Sweet Potato Salad

Serves: 2 / Serving Size: 5 ounces chicken, 1 cup potatoes, 2 cups salad

3/4 pound sweet potatoes
2 tablespoons balsamic vinegar
1 tablespoon Dijon mustard
1 tablespoon plus 2 teaspoons olive oil, divided
2 tablespoons water
Salt and freshly ground black pepper, to taste
1/2 cup diced red onion
1/2 cup sliced celery
3/4 pound boneless, skinless chicken breasts
1/2 small head romaine lettuce, washed and torn into bite-size pieces
1/2 cup chopped fresh parsley
1 medium tomato, cut into wedges

1. Peel potatoes and cut into 1/2-inch pieces. Place in a medium-size nonstick saucepan and cover with cold water. Cover with a lid and boil 10 minutes or until potatoes are cooked.

2. Whisk the vinegar and mustard together in a medium-size bowl. Whisk in 1 tablespoon oil and the water. Add salt and pepper to taste. Add the onion and celery and toss well.

3. When potatoes are cooked, drain and add (while still warm) to the bowl of dressing. Add salt and pepper to taste. Toss well. Set aside.

4. Cut chicken into 1/2-inch pieces (about the same size as the potatoes). In the same saucepan used for the potatoes, heat the 2 remaining teaspoons oil over medium-high heat. Sauté chicken 3–4 minutes. A meat

thermometer inserted into chicken should read 165°F. Sprinkle with salt and pepper to taste. Add to the potatoes while still warm, and mix.

5. Place a layer of lettuce leaves on a serving platter. Spoon salad onto lettuce. Sprinkle with parsley. Place tomatoes around edge of platter.

*Exchanges/Food Choices: 3 starch, 1 vegetable, 4 1/2 lean protein, 1 1/2 fat*
*Per serving: Calories 530, Calories from Fat 150, Total Fat 17 g, Saturated Fat 2.5 g,*
*Monounsaturated Fat 10 g, Cholesterol 125 mg, Sodium 410 mg, Potassium 1830 mg,*
*Total Carbohydrate 50 g, Dietary Fiber 10 g, Sugars 15 g, Protein 44 g, Phosphorus 530 mg*

## Shopping List:

3/4 pound sweet potatoes
1 jar Dijon mustard
1 red onion
1 bunch celery
3/4 pound boneless, skinless chicken breasts
1 small head romaine lettuce
1 bunch parsley
1 medium tomato

## Staples:

Balsamic vinegar
Olive oil
Salt and black peppercorns

## Helpful Hint:

■ Any type of waxy potatoes, such as yellow or new potatoes, can be used.

# Cock-a-Leekie Soup

*This is a Scottish peasant soup with recipes dating back to the 16th century. The traditional recipe takes about 1 1/2 hours to make. This is a shortened version that has all of the flavors of the original without the long cooking time.*

## Countdown:

- Prepare ingredients.
- Make soup.

## Cock-a-Leekie Soup

Serves: 2 / Serving Size: 2 cups soup (including 5 ounces chicken)

2 teaspoons olive oil
1 1/2 pounds skinless, bone-in chicken legs
1 cup sliced carrots
1 cup sliced celery
2 large leeks, cleaned and sliced (about 3 cups)
2 cups fat-free, low-sodium chicken stock
2 cups water
1/4 cup quick pearl barley
1/4 teaspoon dried thyme
Salt and freshly ground black pepper, to taste
2 tablespoons chopped parsley (optional)

1. Heat oil in a large saucepan and add chicken legs, carrots, and celery. Sauté 10 minutes, turning the chicken over several times to brown all sides.

2. Add the leeks, chicken stock, water, barley, and thyme to the saucepan. Bring to a simmer, cover with a lid, and cook 10 minutes or until barley is cooked.

3. Remove chicken to a cutting board. A meat thermometer inserted into chicken should read 170°F. Cut the chicken meat from the leg and divide between 2 large soup bowls.

4. Ladle the soup into the bowls. Add salt and pepper to taste. Sprinkle parsley on top (optional).

*Exchanges/Food Choices: 2 starch, 2 vegetable, 5 lean protein, 1 fat*
*Per serving: Calories 470, Calories from Fat 120, Total Fat 13 g, Saturated Fat 2.5 g, Monounsaturated Fat 6 g, Cholesterol 160 mg, Sodium 420 mg, Potassium 1280 mg, Total Carbohydrate 46 g, Dietary Fiber 9 g, Sugars 9 g, Protein 44 g, Phosphorus 520 mg*

## Shopping List:

1 1/2 pounds skinless, bone-in chicken legs
1 package sliced carrots
1 bunch celery
2 large leeks
1 package quick pearl barley
1 bottle dried thyme
1 bunch parsley (optional)

## Staples:

Olive oil
Fat-free, low-sodium chicken stock
Salt and black peppercorns

## Helpful Hints:

- Slice vegetables in food processor fitted with slicing blade.
- To clean leeks, slice them in half lengthwise and rinse under cold running water.
- Make sure your bottles of dried herbs and spices are less than 6 months old.

## Shop Smart:

- Look for fat-free, low-sodium chicken stock or broth with 20 calories per cup and about 150 mg sodium per cup.

# Garlic-Chicken Soup with Sesame-Parmesan Crostini

*Garlic lovers, this soup is for you! Garlic-laced mayonnaise spread on a floating crostini adds an extra punch to the soup. Cooking chicken legs on the bone gives extra texture to this dish.*

## Countdown:

- Start chicken and vegetables.
- Prepare remaining ingredients.
- While soup cooks, make garlic mayonnaise and toast.

## Garlic-Chicken Soup with Sesame-Parmesan Crostini

Serves: 2 / Serving Size: 2 1/4 cups soup (including 5 ounces chicken), 1 slice bread

2 teaspoons canola oil
1 1/2 pounds skinless, bone-in chicken legs
1 cup sliced onion
1 cup sliced celery
Salt and freshly ground black pepper, to taste
2 tablespoons flour
2 cups fat-free, low-sodium chicken stock
1 cup water
1/2 teaspoon dried thyme
1/2 pound broccoli florets
4 garlic cloves, crushed, divided
2 slices whole-wheat baguette (about 2 inches in diameter)
2 1/2 tablespoons reduced-fat mayonnaise

1. Heat oil in a large nonstick saucepan or deep skillet. Add the chicken legs, onion, and celery. Sauté chicken 10 minutes, turning the chicken legs over several times.

2. Add flour to the onion and celery in the saucepan. Stir to mix in with the vegetables. Slowly add the chicken stock and water, and stir to thicken the broth. Add the thyme, broccoli, and 2 crushed garlic cloves to the saucepan. Bring to a simmer and cook 5 minutes.

3. While chicken cooks, toast the baguette slices. Then mix the 2 remaining crushed garlic cloves and mayonnaise together. Spread over the toast.

4. Remove chicken to a cutting board. A meat thermometer inserted into chicken should read 170°F. Cut the meat off the bones.

5. Divide the meat between 2 large soup bowls. Ladle the soup into the bowls, and float one piece of toast in each bowl.

*Exchanges/Food Choices: 1 1/2 starch, 1 vegetable, 5 1/2 lean protein, 2 fat*
*Per serving: Calories 470, Calories from Fat 170, Total Fat 19 g, Saturated Fat 3.5 g,*
*Monounsaturated Fat 7 g, Cholesterol 160 mg, Sodium 600 mg, Potassium 1380 mg,*
*Total Carbohydrate 30 g, Dietary Fiber 3 g, Sugars 5 g, Protein 46 g, Phosphorus 600 mg*

## Shopping List:

1 1/2 pounds skinless, bone-in chicken legs
1 bunch celery
1 bottle dried thyme
1/2 pound broccoli florets
1 whole-wheat baguette

## Staples:

Canola oil
Onion
Salt and black peppercorns
Flour
Fat-free, low-sodium chicken stock
Garlic
Reduced-fat mayonnaise

## Helpful Hints:

■ Any type of onion can be used.
■ Look for skinless, bone-in chicken legs, or remove the skin before cooking.
■ Use a saucepan or deep skillet just large enough to fit the chicken legs in one layer.
■ Make sure your bottles of dried herbs and spices are less than 6 months old.

## Shop Smart:

■ Look for fat-free, low-sodium chicken stock or broth with 20 calories per cup and about 150 mg sodium per cup.

# Alphabetical Index

# K

Kung Pao Chicken with Chinese Noodles, 98–99

# L

Lemon-Pepper Chicken with Carrot and Zucchini Cannellini Beans, 22–23

# M

Mango Salsa Pan-Roasted Chicken and Hot Peanut Rice, 24–25

Mediterranean Chicken with Sautéed Fresh Corn, 76–77

Mexican Orange Chicken with Green Pepper Rice, 58–59

Moroccan Spiced Chicken with Spinach and Lentils, 78–79

Mu Shu Chicken Wrap with Chinese Egg Noodles, 100–101

# O

Orange-Honey Chicken with Garlic Zucchini and Grape Tomatoes, 26–27

Oven-Fried Chicken with Creamed Corn and Lima Beans, 28–29

# P

Pecan-Crusted, Honey-Glazed Chicken with Rosemary-Garlic Cannellini Beans, 30–31

Penne Puttanesca with Italian Salad, 80–81

Puerto Rican Chicken and Rice, 60–61

# R

Rosemary-Garlic Chicken with Crunchy Cucumber Rice, 82–83

# S

Sangria-Braised Pulled Chicken Sliders with Quick Slaw, 32–33

Savory Sage Chicken with Zucchini and Tomato Rice, 34–35

Sesame Chicken with Snow Peas and Rice, 102–103

Sloppy Joes with Dipping Veggies, 116–117

Southwestern Chicken Burgers with Tortilla Salad, 36–37

Spiced Chicken with Tangerine Sauce and Apricot Couscous, 84–85

Stir-Fried Diced Chicken with Cucumbers and Brown Rice, 104–105

Stout-Soused Chicken with Potatoes and Leeks, 38–39

Sun-Dried Tomato and Chicken Sandwich, 118–119

Sweet and Sour Meatballs with Egg Noodles and Peas, 40–41

# W

Walnut-Crusted Chicken with Tomato and Bean Salad, 42–43

Wasabi Chicken with Pan-Roasted Ginger, Corn, and Snow Peas, 106–107

# Subject Index

## A

All American

  Almond-Maple Chicken with Hot Pepper Succotash, 2–3

  Cajun Chicken and Caramelized Onion Rice, 4–5

  Chicken in Red Wine with Parsley Noodles, 8–9

  Chicken in Sherry-Mushroom Sauce with Herbed Quinoa, 6–7

  Creole Chicken with Rice, 10–11

  Devil's Chicken with Sautéed Garlic Potatoes, 12–13

  Dilled Chicken Parcels with Parsley Rice, 14–15

  Fresh Herbed Chicken with Red Potatoes and Green Beans, 16–17

  Horseradish-Encrusted Chicken with Garlic Sweet Potatoes and Sugar Snap Peas, 18–19

  Hot Pepper Chicken with Sweet Pepper Potatoes, 20–21

  Lemon-Pepper Chicken with Carrot and Zucchini Cannellini Beans, 22–23

  Mango Salsa Pan-Roasted Chicken and Hot Peanut Rice, 24–25

  Orange-Honey Chicken with Garlic Zucchini and Grape Tomatoes, 26–27

  Oven-Fried Chicken with Creamed Corn and Lima Beans, 28–29

  Pecan-Crusted, Honey-Glazed Chicken with Rosemary-Garlic Cannellini Beans, 30–31

  Sangria-Braised Pulled Chicken Sliders with Quick Slaw, 32–33

  Savory Sage Chicken with Zucchini and Tomato Rice, 34–35

  Southwestern Chicken Burgers with Tortilla Salad, 36–37

  Stout-Soused Chicken with Potatoes and Leeks, 38–39

  Sweet and Sour Meatballs with Egg Noodles and Peas, 40–41

  Walnut-Crusted Chicken with Tomato and Bean Salad, 42–43

All-American Chicken Salad Supper, 122–123

allspice, 124–125

Almond-Maple Chicken with Hot Pepper Succotash, 2–3

apricot/apricot jam, 84–85, 92–93

arugula, 80–81, 118–119

Asian/Indian

  Chicken Satay with Thai Peanut Sauce and Broccoli Rice, 90–91

  Curry-Kissed Chicken with Rice and Carrots, 92–93

  "Dead Easy" Chicken with Chinese Rice, 94–95

  Japanese Barbecued Chicken and Mushrooms with Sesame Rice, 96–97

  Kung Pao Chicken with Chinese Noodles, 98–99

  Mu Shu Chicken Wrap with Chinese Egg Noodles, 100–101

  Sesame Chicken with Snow Peas and Rice, 102–103

  Stir-Fried Diced Chicken with Cucumbers and Brown Rice, 104–105

  Wasabi Chicken with Pan-Roasted Ginger, Corn, and Snow Peas, 106–107

## B

Barbecued Chicken Roll with Peppery Bean Salad, 110–111

barley, 128–129

basil, 64–65, 80–81, 118–119

bean

  Barbecued Chicken Roll with Peppery Bean Salad, 110–111

  black, 48–49, 124–125

  cannellini, 22–23, 30–31

Chicken-Mushroom Quesadillas with Corn and Black Bean Salad, 48–49
Fresh Herbed Chicken with Red Potatoes and Green Beans, 16–17
Great Northern, 42–43
green, 12–13, 16–17
kidney, 110–111
Lemon-Pepper Chicken with Carrot and Zucchini Cannellini Beans, 22–23
lima, 2–3, 28–29
Oven-Fried Chicken with Creamed Corn and Lima Beans, 28–29
Pecan-Crusted, Honey-Glazed Chicken with Rosemary-Garlic Cannellini Beans, 30–31
refried, xii, 50–51
Walnut-Crusted Chicken with Tomato and Bean Salad, 42–43
bean sprout, 94–95
bibb lettuce, 70–71
blueberry, 122–123
Brazilian-Style Chicken and Quinoa, 46–47
bread
baguette, 130–131
hamburger roll, 36–37, 110–111, 116–117
multi-grain, 118–119, 122–123
pita, xi, 112–113
slider roll, 32–33
broccoli, 90–91, 98–99, 116–117, 130–131

# C

cabbage, 32–33, 100–101
Cajun Chicken and Caramelized Onion Rice, 4–5
caper, 66–67
Caribbean. See Latin and Caribbean
Caribbean Chicken Salad, 124–125
carrot, 22–23, 92–93, 116–117, 128–129
catsup, xii, 116–117
celery, 10–11, 116–117, 126–129

cheese, 64–65, 72–73, 80–81, 130–131
chicken, ground, xii
Chicken Enchiladas with Esquites, 50–51
Chicken in Red Wine with Parsley Noodles, 8–9
Chicken in Sherry-Mushroom Sauce with Herbed Quinoa, 6–7
Chicken Parmesan with Basil Linguine, 64–65
Chicken Piccata with Spaghettini, 66–67
Chicken Pita Pocket with Greek Salad, 112–113
Chicken Ragout with Mushroom Rice, 68–69
Chicken Satay with Thai Peanut Sauce and Broccoli Rice, 90–91
Chicken Tricolore with Spicy Potatoes, 70–71
Chicken-Mushroom Quesadillas with Corn and Black Bean Salad, 48–49
Chicken–Sweet Potato Salad, 126–127
Chimichurri Chicken with Red Pepper and Tomato Penne, 52–53
Chimichurri sauce, xii, 52–53
Chinese five-spice powder, 94–95
cilantro, 60–61
cinnamon/cinnamon stick, 32–33, 78–79
Cock-a-Leekie Soup, 128–129
coconut/coconut milk, xi, 46–47, 56–57
condiment, x. See also under specific type
cooking tips, ix, x
corn, 2–3, 28–29, 48–51, 76–77, 106–107, 112–113
couscous, 84–85
Creole Chicken with Rice, 10–11
cucumber, 74–75, 82–83, 104–105, 112–113
cumin, 46–47, 78–79, 84–85
Curried Chicken Salad Wrap, 114–115
Curry-Kissed Chicken with Rice and Carrots, 92–93

# D

"Dead Easy" Chicken with Chinese Rice, 94–95

Devil's Chicken with Sautéed Garlic Potatoes, 12–13

Dilled Chicken Parcels with Parsley Rice, 14–15

# E

Esquites, 50–51

# F

Fresh Herbed Chicken with Red Potatoes and Green Beans, 16–17

frozen ingredients, x

# G

garlic, 12–13, 18–19, 26–27, 30–31, 82–83, 104–105, 130–131

Garlic-Chicken Soup with Sesame-Parmesan Crostini, 130–131

ginger, 98–99, 102–103, 106–107

Gorgonzola Chicken Scaloppini with Fresh Linguine and Sweet Pimentos, 72–73

grain, x. See also under specific type

Grilled Chicken with Greek Tomato Salad and Brown Rice, 74–75

# H

helpful hints, ix

Henry IV, ix

herb, x, 6–7, 16–17, 76–77

Herbes de Provence, 76–77

hoisin sauce, 98–101, 104–105

Hom, Ken, 94

honey, 20–21, 26–27, 30–31, 102–103

horseradish, 18–19, 122–123

Horseradish-Encrusted Chicken with Garlic Sweet Potatoes and Sugar Snap Peas, 18–19

Hot Pepper Chicken with Sweet Pepper Potatoes, 20–21

hot pepper jelly, 2–3, 42–43

# I

Indian. *See* Asian/Indian

Island Chicken and Papaya with Pigeon Peas and Rice, 54–55

Italian Meat Loaf with Hot Pepper Lentils, 86–88

# J

Jamaican Jerk Chicken and Quinoa with Coconut and Spinach, 56–57

Japanese Barbecued Chicken and Mushrooms with Sesame Rice, 96–97

jerking, 56–57

# K

ketchup, xii, 116–117

Kung Pao Chicken with Chinese Noodles, 98–99

# L

Latin and Caribbean

Brazilian-Style Chicken and Quinoa, 46–47

Chicken Enchiladas with Esquites, 50–51

Chicken-Mushroom Quesadillas with Corn and Black Bean Salad, 48–49

Chimichurri Chicken with Red Pepper and Tomato Penne, 52–53

Island Chicken and Papaya with Pigeon Peas and Rice, 54–55

Jamaican Jerk Chicken and Quinoa with Coconut and Spinach, 56–57

Mexican Orange Chicken with Green Pepper Rice, 58–59

Puerto Rican Chicken and Rice, 60–61

leek, 38–39, 128–129

lemon/lemon juice, 22–23, 66–67

Lemon-Pepper Chicken with Carrot and Zucchini Cannellini Beans, 22–23

lentil, 78–79, 86–88

lettuce, 70–71, 100–101, 112–113, 126–127

# Q

# R

# S

Sun-Dried Tomato and Chicken
Sandwich, 118–119
Walnut-Crusted Chicken with Tomato
and Bean Salad, 42–43
tortilla/tortilla chip, xi, 36–37, 48–51,
114–115

# V

vegetable, x, 116–117. *See also under
specific type*

# W

Walnut-Crusted Chicken with Tomato
and Bean Salad, 42–43
Wasabi Chicken with Pan-Roasted
Ginger, Corn, and Snow Peas,
106–107
wine, 8–9, 32–33, 66–67

# Z

zucchini, 22–23, 26–27, 34–35